FAST FACTS

Indispensable Guides to Clinical Practice

Endometriosis

Hossam Abdalla
Director of the Fertility and Endocrinology Centre, The Lister Hospital, London, UK

Botros Rizk
Associate Professor, Department of Obstetrics & Gynecology and Director of the Division of Reproductive Endocrinology, University of South Alabama, Mobile, Alabama, USA

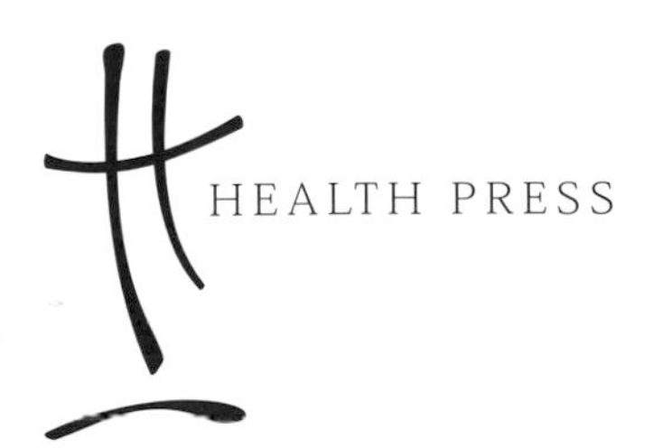

Oxford

Fast Facts – Endometriosis
First published 1998

Elizabeth House, Queen Street, Abingdon, Oxford, UK OX14 3JR

Tel: +44 (0)1235 523233
Fax: +44 (0)1235 523238

A CIP catalogue record for this title is available from the British Library.

ISBN 1-899541-22-5

Library of Congress
Cataloging-in-Publication Data

Abdalla, H. (Hossam)
Fast Facts – Endometriosis/
Hossam Abdalla, Botros Rizk

Designed by Hinton Chaundy Design Partnership, Thame, UK

Illustrations by Dee McLean and Jane Fallows,
MeDee Art, London, UK

Printed by Sterling Press, Wellingborough, UK

Glossary 4

Introduction 5

Epidemiology and pathogenesis 7

Endometriosis and infertility 22

Diagnosis 27

Medical treatment 35

Surgical treatment 41

Treatment of associated infertility 47

Assisted reproductive technology and endometriosis 52

Extrapelvic endometriosis 56

Recurrent endometriosis 61

Adenomyosis 64

The doctor/patient partnership 68

Key references 70

Index 72

Glossary

adhesiolysis: separation/removal of adhesions

adnexal masses: enlarged parts of the Fallopian tubes or ovaries

amenorrhoea: absence of menstruation

anovulation: lack of ovulation

blebs: blister-like lumps filled with fluid

dizygotic: non-identical (e.g. twins)

dyschezia: painful defecation

dysmenorrhoea: pain before and during menstruation

dyspareunia: painful sexual intercourse

dysuria: pain on passing urine

endometrial atrophy: pseudopregnancy

endometrioma: tumour of abnormally placed endometrium

endometriosis scores: method of evaluating the disease

fecundity rate: fertility rating

GnRH: gonadotrophin-releasing hormone

GnRH analogues: superstimulate the pituitary gland to make more GnRH

GnRH antagonists: stop the production of GnRH

haematuria: blood in the urine

hirsutism: excessive growth of hair on face and body

hypermenorrhoea: heavy menstrual bleeding

hyperplasia: abnormal increase in tissue cells

hyperprolactinaemia: abnormally high production of the hormone prolactin

implantation: penetration of and attachment to the lining of the womb

macrophages: scavenging cells of the immune system

mesothelium: lining cells of the peritoneum, pleura and other body parts

metaplasia: abnormal change in tissue as a result of change in cells

monozygotic: identical (e.g. twins)

oestradiol: major female sex hormone produced by the ovary. Also used as a drug to control menopausal symptoms

oligomenorrhoea: abnormally infrequent periods

oophorectomy: surgical removal of ovaries

peritoneal fluid: lubricant secreted by the peritoneum

prostaglandins: hormone-like substances that react to body change (e.g. influencing blood clotting, inducing abortion, causing muscle contraction)

retrograde menstruation: menstrual blood that stays in the body

superovulation: production of more than one or two ova at one time

synthetic progestogens: drugs chemically and pharmacologically similar to natural hormone progesterone

uterine fibroids: benign tumours growing in the uterus wall

Introduction

Endometriosis is one of the most common gynaecological conditions in women of reproductive age, yet it remains one of the most complicated and baffling. It is estimated that over 5 million women in the USA have endometriosis. Sufferers make up a sizeable proportion of those attending gynaecological practices, whether seeking help for infertility or because the condition has become chronic with disabling effects. Although it is not easy to determine how prevalent the disease is among the general population (at present, it can only be confirmed by laparoscopy or laparotomy), there are indications that it is increasing. One factor determining prevalence could be the considerable delay between the onset of pain symptoms and the surgical diagnosis – in the UK it is 8 years, in the USA 11.7 years.

In addition to the physical effects of the disease, the psychological impact of endometriosis is also a cause for concern. Every practising family physician and gynaecologist should be aware of the feelings of frustration and consequent depression experienced by women with endometriosis.

On numerous occasions women have been referred to psychiatrists as 'mental cases', a 'psychologizing of endometriosis' that represents the failure of gynaecologists to diagnose the condition. In one clinic, out of 850 laparoscopies performed in patients with pain of 6 months' duration or longer, histologically proven endometriosis or adhesions were found in 92%. After treatment, their psychological profiles returned to near normal – when endometriosis is removed, pain is successfully cured.

Gynaecologists must not allow frustrated or ill-informed colleagues to dismiss patients rather than diagnose and treat them; they should be encouraged to refer them to specialists who can.

Though the disease has been known about for more than a century, it remains a challenge to gynaecologists and family physicians. *Fast Facts – Endometriosis* presents healthcare professionals with the latest information to enable the patient to be treated with due consideration and speed.

CHAPTER 1

Epidemiology and pathogenesis

The incidence of endometriosis remains unknown as the disease is usually recorded as part of another investigation, such as for infertility or chronic pain in the abdomen or pelvis, or while undergoing another procedure such as sterilization. There are conflicting data and it is unclear whether the disease is overdiagnosed or underdiagnosed. Many factors could account for the variation in the estimates of prevalence of endometriosis drawn from different investigations.

Prevalence

Estimates in the USA are often based on surgical records and those of hospitalized patients. In 1980, among women aged 15–44 years, 6.3% of first diagnosis and 6.9% of all diagnoses for genitourinary problems were due to endometriosis (National Centre for Health Statistics).

Between 1988 and 1990 the US National Hospital Discharge Survey, covering over 5 million gynaecological diagnoses, put endometriosis as first diagnosis in 11.2% of women.

US Army records (1980–85) show that endometriosis was diagnosed in 6.2% of women undergoing gynaecological surgery. Another review from Houston, Texas, put the prevalence of endometriosis at 10.3%.

Smaller surgical case reports show a range of findings: when laparoscopy was performed for pelvic pain, a prevalence rate of 4–80% was reported for endometriosis compared with 2–80% for infertility. Endometriosis was reported in 1–4% of around 10 000 women undergoing tubal ligation.

In the UK, endometriosis was noted in 21% of women being investigated for infertility and in 6% being sterilized. For those with chronic abdominal pain, the incidence of endometriosis was 15%; among those having abdominal hysterectomy, it was 25%.

Houston and co-authors reviewed the medical records of white residents of Rochester, Minnesota, USA, from 1970 to 1979, to find newly diagnosed cases of endometriosis. They had four diagnostic groups:

- histologically confirmed disease
- visualization of disease during surgery

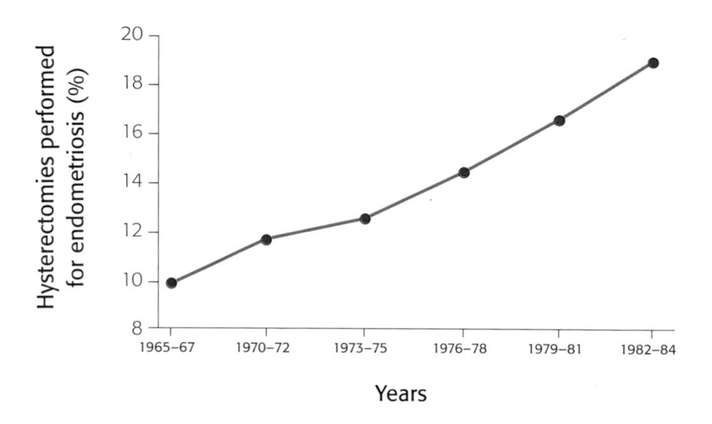

Figure 1.1 Proportion of hysterectomies performed in the USA for endometriosis. Reproduced with permission from Nezhat CR *et al.*, eds. *Endometriosis: Advanced Management and Surgical Techniques.* New York: Springer-Verlag, 1995.

- clinically probable diagnosis based on pain and positive examination
- clinically possible diagnosis based on examination alone.

From these data, the authors concluded a prevalence of between 2.5% and 3.3% – assuming that the endometriosis had an average duration of 10 years. However, should the duration be 25 years, the prevalence rate would be 6.2–8.2%. As there is known to be considerable delay in the diagnosis (i.e. between the onset of pain symptoms and the surgical confirmation), prevalence rates should take this into account.

Kjerulff and colleagues used the self-reporting method (US Health Interview Survey, 1984–1992), asking a random sample aged 18–50 years about their gynaecological problems in the previous year. In the 341 617 women surveyed, the prevalence of endometriosis was 6.9/1000, while that of menstrual disorders was 53/1000. The authors acknowledged that these reported rates could be underestimates because many respondents were too embarrassed to answer personal questions. Others had not reported their symptoms to a physician; some had forgotten about them.

Changes in prevalence. Gynaecological surgery for endometriosis has increased over the last three decades (Figure 1.1). In 1965, approximately 130 000 hysterectomies were performed for endometriosis in the USA compared with 390 000 in 1984. Although the general trend was an increase in the number of hysterectomies performed during this period, the increase in those carried out for endometriosis (Figure 1.2) was unmatched by any other condition. As there is more diagnosis today, the reported prevalence is increasing.

Risk factors

A number of factors appear to increase the risk of endometriosis (Table 1.1).

Race appears to be an important factor affecting susceptibility to endometriosis. The incidence of endometriosis is thought to be higher in Japanese women than white women. Although some studies have suggested that white women are more likely to develop endometriosis than black women, the differences are insignificant once confounding variables are taken into account.

Hereditary factors. A genetic or familial tendency to endometriosis has been repeatedly reported. Sampson and colleagues found endometriosis in 5.8% of siblings of patients and 8.1% of their mothers. Overall, about 7% of all first-degree relatives were affected compared with 1% of the female relatives of the patient's husband.

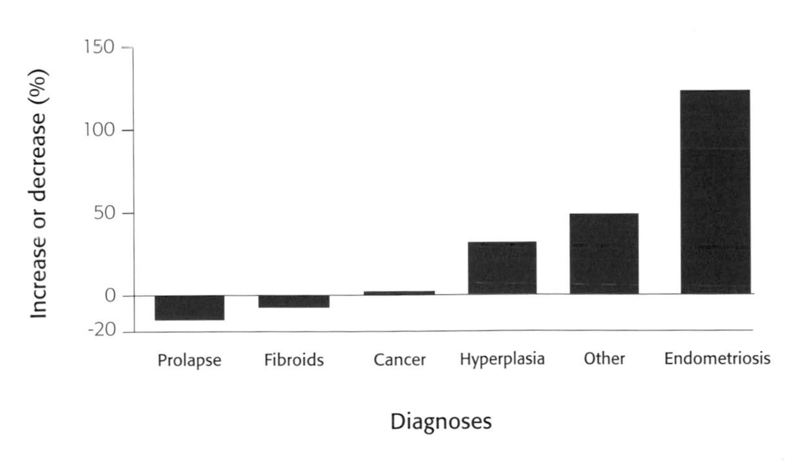

Figure 1.2 Changes in the indications for hysterectomy in the USA between 1965 and 1984. Reproduced with permission from Nezhat CR *et al.*, eds. *Endometriosis: Advanced Management and Surgical Techniques.* New York: Springer-Verlag, 1995.

TABLE 1.1
Risk factors

Increased risk
• Japanese race
• Family history
• Oestrogen status
• Age 30–44 years
• Increased menstrual flow and decreased cycle length
• Environmental factors
• Alcohol
• Increased peripheral body fat
Decreased risk
• Current and recent contraceptive users
• Current IUD users, possibly
• Smokers

The disease has been shown to be more common among monozygotic twin sisters of patients with endometriosis compared with dizygotic sisters. It also appears to be more severe in women with a first-degree relative with endometriosis. Twins with endometriosis have a higher degree of bilateral and early onset disease.

Hormonal. There is strong circumstantial evidence that endometriosis is dependent on steroid hormones. The disease has not been reported in premenarchal girls and the rare cases in post-menopausal women have been related to hormone replacement therapy (HRT). Thus, conditions that alter oestrogen status may influence the incidence of endometriosis.

Age. A positive relationship between endometriosis and age has been observed, with a peak at 40 years of age. Compared with women aged 25–29 years, the risk of endometriosis is increased among women aged 30–44 years.

Environmental. Links between endometriosis and chemical substances present in everyday life have been shown. Synthetic oestrogens include a non-steroidal hormone agonist and phenolic impurities found in some dyes and polycarbonate plastics. In addition, many industrial chemicals, agricultural pesticides and metabolites have oestrogenic activity when chlorinated.

Tetrachlorodibenzo-P-dioxin (TCDD) is the prototype. Although contact with TCDD and dioxin-like substances can be occupational or accidental, exposure is generally through eating foods that have been subjected to the atmospheric effects of natural events, such as volcanic eruption, forest and wood-burning fires, or the by-products of manufacturing (Table 1.2). WHO currently recommends that the intake of TCCD should be limited to 10 pg/kg body weight/day.

TABLE 1.2

Sources of dioxins

- Waste incineration
- Many types of metal production
- Fossil fuel and petrol refining
- Bleaching in the manufacture of white paper

Socio-economic status. Only one of the studies examining the relationship between endometriosis and socio-economic status has reported a positive association. The suggestion that endometriosis is a disease of white, middle class, career-orientated, egocentric and perfectionist women has no scientific basis.

Menstrual and reproductive history. There is an association between endometriosis and certain menstrual patterns. The risk is greater in women who have:

- increased menstrual pain (Figure 1.3)
- increased duration of flow (Figure 1.4)
- decreased cycle length (Figure 1.4)
- uterine abnormalities that occlude normal menstrual flow
- had an early menarche.

These factors, together with the fact that women today have a greater number of menses than their Victorian counterparts, might partly explain the apparent increased incidence of the disease.

Generally, risk of endometriosis is decreased in women who have previously been pregnant for any length of time. The longer the pregnancy, the more protective the effect, though

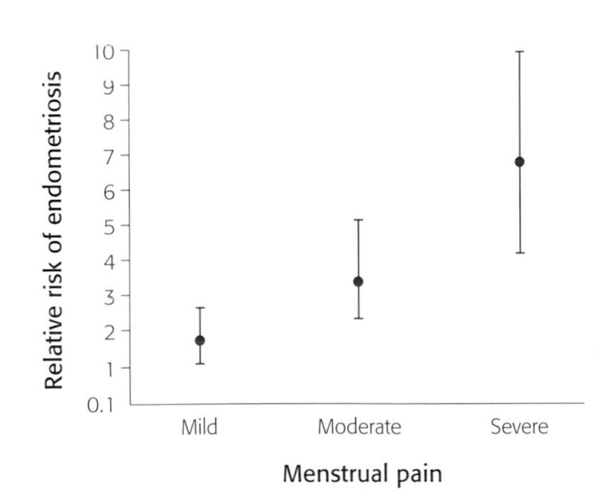

Figure 1.3 The relative risk of endometriosis is greater in women who experience more menstrual pain.

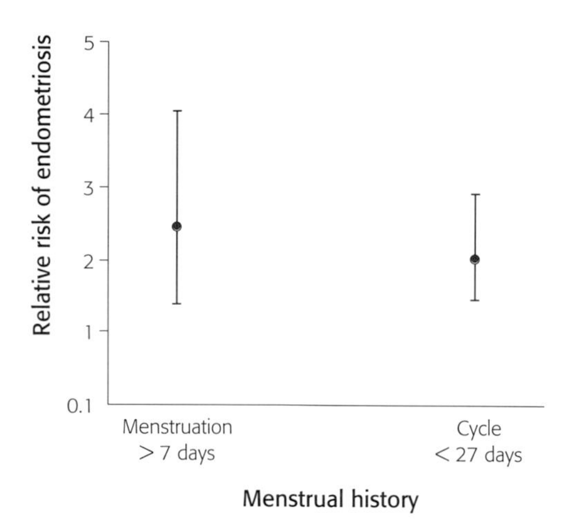

Figure 1.4 The relative risk of endometriosis is greater in women with increased duration of menstrual flow and decreased cycle length.

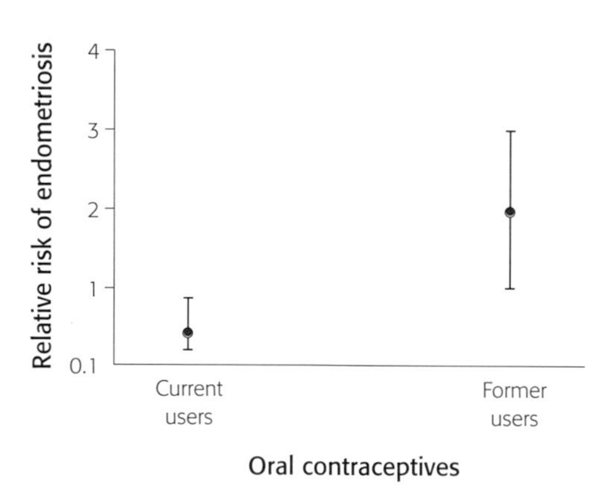

Figure 1.5 The risk of endometriosis is increased in women who have used oral contraceptives 25–48 months previously, but is decreased in current or recent users.

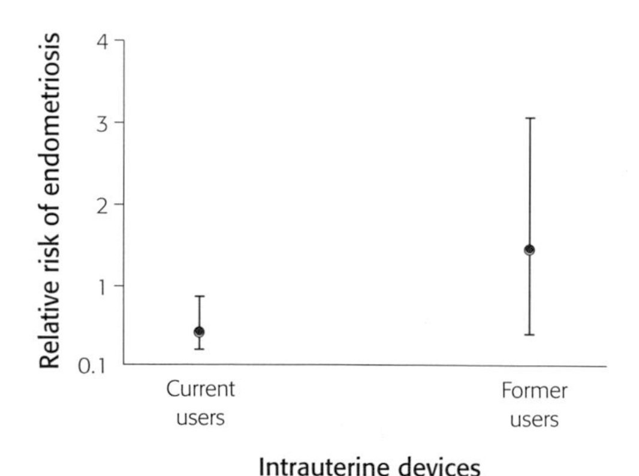

Figure 1.6 The risk of endometriosis is increased in women who have used the intrauterine device 49–72 months previously, but is decreased in current users.

it appears to wane as the years since the last birth increase. A case control study showed the odds ratio for endometriosis was 4.5 in those who had not given birth in 10 years, compared with women of a similar age who had had a baby in the previous 5 years.

Contraceptive use. In the only population-based cohort study conducted to date, Vessey and colleagues used the Oxford Family Planning Association study data to look for a relationship between contraceptive use and endometriosis (all cases were confirmed by laparoscopy). The authors reported that those currently or recently using oral contraceptives were less likely to have endometriosis than those who had used oral contraceptives 25–48 months previously (Figure 1.5); there was no association between the disease and the duration of oral contraceptive use. It appears that oral contraceptives may mask endometriosis and its symptoms, and these only emerge after oral contraceptives are discontinued.

In a study comparing women currently or recently using the intrauterine device (0–12 months), former users (49–72 months) and women who had never used an IUD, the risk was increased in the former users but decreased in current users compared with those who had never used an IUD (Figure 1.6).

No association was found between diaphragm use and endometriosis.

Alcohol. Several of the gynaecological symptoms of women with endometriosis are also found in women who abuse alcohol or are dependent on it. Endometriosis patients have higher scores than control patients on the Michigan Alcoholism Screening Test and consume more alcohol on a yearly basis.

The link between social and behavioural factors, alcohol and infertility was studied by Grodstein and co-workers: the odds ratio for endometriosis was 1.7 for moderate drinkers and 1.8 for heavy drinkers compared with infertile women who did not drink.

Caffeine. Grodstein looked at caffeine use in 1050 women with primary infertility and in 3833 women who had recently given birth. Those who drank more coffee were found to have a significant increase in risk of infertility as a result of tubal disease or endometriosis. This effect, however, seems more likely to be a result of the lifestyle of patients with endometriosis. Further epidemiological studies are required to evaluate these findings.

Smoking. Studies investigating the effects of smoking on reproductive function have produced conflicting results. Vessey *et al.* showed no association between endometriosis and smoking. Cramer, in a study of heavy smokers (> 1 pack of cigarettes/day) who had started to smoke before 17 years of age, showed an inverse relationship between endometriosis and smoking, and an increased risk of infertility (odds ratio = 0.5, 95% confidence intervals 0.3–0.9).

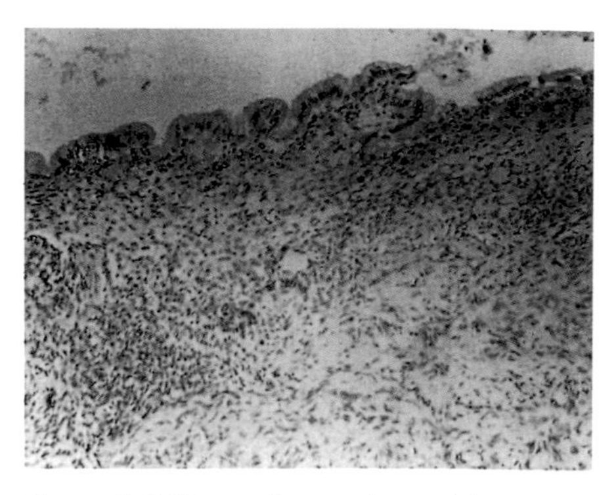

Figure 1.7 Biopsy of an endometrial cyst showing superficial endometrial tissue growing on the ovarian cortex. Reproduced with permission from Nezhat CR *et al.,* eds. *Endometriosis: Advanced Management and Surgical Techniques.* New York: Springer-Verlag, 1995.

Smokers are relatively oestrogen deficient, as smoking appears to alter oestrogen metabolism. They have an earlier natural menopause, a lower risk of endometrial cancer, an increased risk of osteoporotic fractures, and a reduced risk of uterine fibroids, endometriosis and benign breast disease, compared with non-smokers.

Dioxins have been reported in cigarette smoke. It is estimated that someone smoking 1 pack/day takes in about 4.3 pg of polychlorinated dibenzodioxins/kg body weight/day. Dioxin exposure should, therefore, be added to the adverse effects of smoking that may increase the risk of infertility. Such effects would outweigh any potential benefits relating to the risk of endometriosis.

Height, weight and body mass. In a study of body fat distribution (n = 176), after adjusting for age, body mass index, parity, age at menarche and intensity of menstrual flow, the risk of endometriosis was shown to be greater in women under 30 years of age with more peripheral body fat than those with more centralized fat. The lack of an effect in older women may be due to a progressive increase in waist circumference with age. This study was small and limited, but the authors' conclusion that greater peripheral body fat may be related to higher oestrogen levels is consistent with the notion that endometriosis depends on oestrogen.

Pathogenesis

Endometriosis is defined as the presence of tissue histologically similar to endometrium outside the uterine cavity (Figure 1.7). 'Endometriosis externa' is used to describe endometriosis outside the uterus. This is most commonly found in the pelvis, but may also occur in the abdominal cavity, the pleura and, very rarely, in the brain and eyes (Figure 1.8). 'Endometriosis interna' describes endometriosis in the uterine myometrium – it is also known as adenomyosis (see Chapter 10).

Although the pathogenesis of endometriosis is complex and still incompletely understood, a number of theories have been developed (Table 1.3).

Implantation theory. This depends on three conditions:

- that retrograde menstruation occurs
- that menstrual blood contains viable endometrial cells
- that the endometrial cells adhere to the peritoneum with subsequent implantation and proliferation.

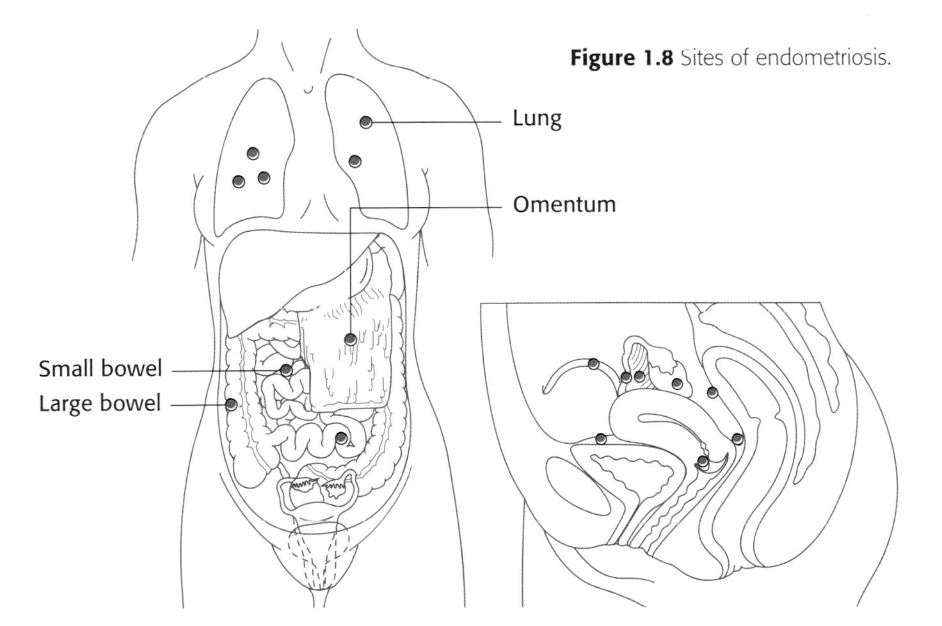

Figure 1.8 Sites of endometriosis.

Sampson's monumental work from Albany, New York, established the theory in the 1920s. It is clear from the source documents that he also described vascular dissemination and direct invasion. He suggested that blood from the uterine cavity at the time of menstruation initiated endometriosis, and his observations were supported by several human and animal models.

TABLE 1.3

Theories of pathogenesis

Implantation

- Retrograde menstruation
- Lymphatic dissemination
- Vascular dissemination
- Direct invasion
- Uterotubal

In situ

- Coelomic metaplasia
- Müllerian duct remnants
- Wolffian duct remnants

Induction

- Endometrial-induced metaplasia

Combination

***In-situ* development.** If endometriosis does not occur as a result of retrograde menstruation, three theories propose that it develops *in situ:*

- coelomic metaplasia theory
- Müllerian duct remnant theory
- Wolffian duct remnant theory.

Coelomic metaplasia is an attractive theory that explains the recurrence of endometriosis at all sites, but scientific evidence for it has yet to be established. If the peritoneal mesothelium has the potential to undergo metaplasia, this would be expected to occur in men too. While there are such case reports in men, they all involve the treatment of metastatic prostate cancer with high-dose oestrogen. Furthermore, if endometriosis is to be attributed to coelomic metaplasia, it should occur at sites where there are coelomic membranes, such as the abdomen and thoracic cavities, yet it is rare in the thorax. Finally, if it is similar to metaplasia elsewhere, it should occur with increasing frequency with advancing age. This is not the clinical pattern of endometriosis as there is an abrupt halt when menstruation ceases at menopause. In postmenopausal women, the disease is associated with stimulation of pre-existing endometriosis by oestrogen replacement therapy or endogenous oestrogen production.

Müllerian duct remnant theory. This theory is based on the fact that rudimentary duplications of the Müllerian system might be present in areas adjacent to the Müllerian ducts, allowing cells of Müllerian origin to develop into functioning endometrium.

Wolffian duct remnant theory. This theory is similar to the Müllerian duct remnant theory, but relates to the Wolffian ducts.

Induction theory. Introduced in 1955 by Levander and Normann, this theory is based on the assumption that endometriosis results from differentiation of mesenchymal cells induced by substances released by degenerating endometrium that reach the peritoneal cavity. Other inductive influences, such as gonadal steroids and follicular fluid contents, have been postulated, and strong circumstantial evidence supports the dependency of endometriosis on steroid hormones.

Combination theory. Nisolle and Donnez suggest that peritoneal endometriosis occurs as a result of retrograde implantation, ovarian endometriosis as a result of coelomic metaplasia, and rectovaginal endometriosis develops in the remnants of the Müllerian ducts.

Classification of endometriosis

Various attempts have been made to classify the many and different stages of endometriosis so that the outcome of treatment can be compared with a certain degree of accuracy. The system most widely used today has evolved from the classification originally developed in 1979 by the American Fertility Society (AFS), which is now known as the American Society for Reproductive Medicine (ASRM).

The AFS/ASRM classification (1996) provides a means of recording information about disease morphology (Figure 1.9) along with the use of colour photographs to ensure consistency in describing the disease appearance (endometriosis may have many different appearances).

Ovarian endometriotic cysts. This diagnosis should be confirmed by histology, or by the presence of four significant features:

- cyst diameter less than 12 cm
- adhesions to pelvic side wall and/or broad ligament

Patient's name

Stage I	(Mild)	1 – 5
Stage II	(Moderate)	6 – 15
Stage III	(Severe)	16 – 30
Stage IV	(Extensive)	31 – 54

Total

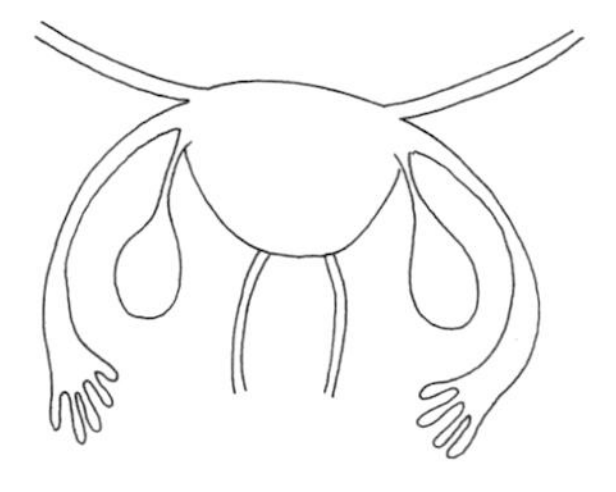

PERITONEUM	ENDOMETRIOSIS	< 1 cm	1–3 cm	> 3 cm
		1	2	3
	ADHESIONS	Filmy	Dense w/partial cul-de-sac obliteration	Dense w/complete cul-de-sac obliteration
		1	2	3
OVARY	ENDOMETRIOSIS	< 1 cm	1–3 cm	> 3 cm or ruptured endometrioma
		2	4	6
		2	4	6
	ADHESIONS	Filmy	Dense w/partial ovarian enclosure	Dense w/complete ovarian enclosure
		2	4	6
		2	4	6
TUBE	ENDOMETRIOSIS	< 1 cm	> 1 cm	Tubal occlusion
		2	4	6
		2	4	6
	ADHESIONS	Filmy	Dense w/tubal distortion	Dense w/tubal enclosure
		2	4	6
		2	4	6

Figure 1.9 Form used for classification of endometriosis. Reproduced with permission from The American Society for Reproductive Medicine.

- endometriosis on the surface of the ovary
- tarry thick chocolate fluid content.

Cul-de-sac obliteration. For this to be complete, no peritoneum should be visible between the uterosacral ligaments.

Morphology of peritoneal and ovarian implants. These should be categorized as red (red, pink and clear lesions), white (white, yellow-brown and peritoneal defects), and black (black and blue lesions). The percentage of involvement of each implant type should be documented.

Stages of endometriosis

Four different stages can be distinguished during the development of the disease (Figure 1.10).

Microscopic endometriosis. If the peritoneum appears to be normal macroscopically, an intraperitoneal lesion may be identified using scanning electron microscopy. This appears as areas of tall and ciliated epithelium, which noticeably replace the mesothelium. Another microscopic appearance is the presence of endometrial glands and stroma under a normal mesothelium.

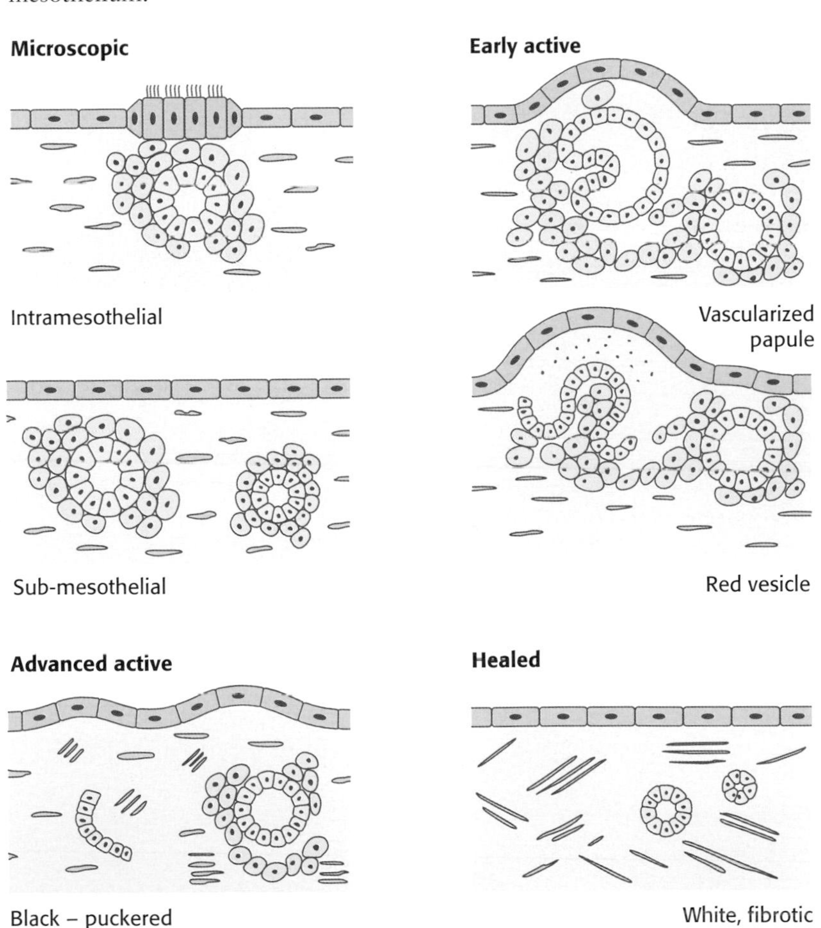

Figure 1.10 Evolution of peritoneal endometriosis.

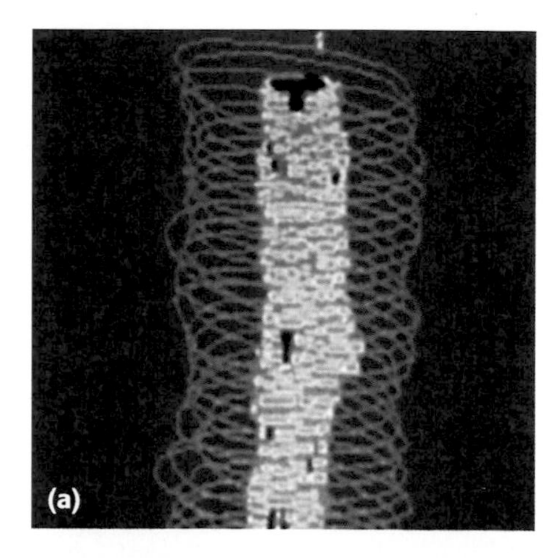

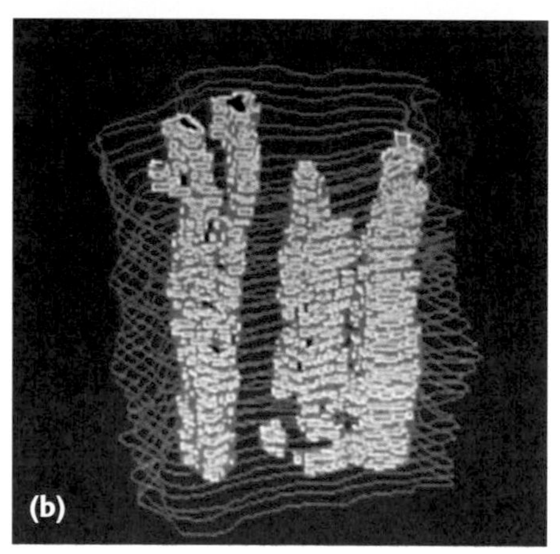

Figure 1.11 Advanced stereographic three-dimensional computer imaging has been used to identify two types of endometrial implant. (a) Regular distribution of the glandular epithelium in the stroma. (b) Glands with ramifications and interconnection of structures. Reproduced with permission from Nezhat CR *et al.*, eds. *Endometriosis: Advanced Management and Surgical Techniques.* New York: Springer-Verlag, 1995.

Early active endometriosis. Polyps, vesicles and papules may be the earliest lesions seen and may appear to be either solid or fluid-filled. They are highly vascular and non-fibrotic. The glands are usually in a proliferative or secretory phase, about one third in phase with the eutopic endometrium. The red haemorrhagic lesions are very active in prostaglandin production.

Advanced active endometriosis. The typical pigmented haemorrhagic and fibrotic endometriotic deposits known as the classic lesions can be seen and are generally out of phase with the eutopic endometrium. As the disease progresses, several stages can coexist at the same site (e.g. early active lesions can disappear or develop into fibrotic lesions).

Healed endometriosis. White scarred lesions are indicative of healed endometriosis. Occasionally, calcified deposits can be seen and active glands can be found among fibrotic end-stage lesions.

Three-dimensional architecture of endometriosis

Though not required by the classification system, Donnez and colleagues have applied advanced stereographic computer technology to identify two types of implants (Figure 1.11). The first, composed of cylinder-like glands without ramifications, shows regular distribution of the glandular epithelia in the stroma. The second type is composed of glands with ramifications; luminal structures are connected to each other and finger-like epithelial structures appear to invade the stroma.

CHAPTER 2

Endometriosis and infertility

While it is easy to understand that advanced and severe endometriosis can cause disruption in the pelvis resulting in mechanical infertility, it is not similarly appreciated that minimal and mild endometriosis could have an impact on a woman conceiving and achieving a live birth. The link between endometriosis and infertility is based on the following observations.

- Endometriosis is prevalent in patients presenting with infertility.
- The fecundity rate in women undergoing donor insemination is significantly reduced if they have endometriosis.
- The induction of experimental endometriosis in animals results in a decrease in the fecundity rate.

There are a number of possible mechanisms that can lead to infertility in patients with mild-to-moderate endometriosis (Table 2.1).

Mechanical pelvic factors

Pelvic endometriosis can cause significant adhesions (Figure 2.1), which can distort the architecture. This interferes with both the release of the oocytes and their transfer into the Fallopian tubes. Other clinical pelvic factors are listed in Table 2.2.

Peritoneal fluid abnormalities

Increase in fluid volume. While several studies have shown an increase in the volume of peritoneal fluid in women with pelvic endometriosis, the correlation between fluid volumes and fertility has not been consistent.

Reduced sperm binding. The peritoneal fluid from women with endometriosis has a negative impact on sperm motility, and sperm binding to the zona pellucida has been shown to be reduced *in vitro*.

Interleukins and tumour necrosis factor. Recent research has shown that interleukins and tumour necrosis factor (TNF) in the peritoneal fluid of endometriosis patients are involved in the inhibition of sperm motility and function, oocyte fertilization and embryo growth.

TABLE 2.1

Possible mechanisms of infertility in patients with mild-to-moderate endometriosis

Changes in peritoneal fluid
• Increase in volume
• Presence of interleukins and tumour necrosis factor
• Increased prostaglandin levels
• Increased number of macrophages
Ovulation disorders
• Anovulation
• Hyperprolactinaemia
• Abnormal follicular genesis
• Premature follicular rupture
• Luteal phase defect
• Luteinized unruptured follicles
Pelvic pain
Immunological abnormalities
• T cells
• Antigen-specific B-cell activation
• Anti-endometrial antibodies
• Non-specific B-cell activation
Spontaneous abortion
Implantation

Prostaglandin levels. Increased prostaglandin levels in the peritoneal fluid of women with endometriosis is another possible explanation of infertility. Prostaglandins alter tube motility and collection of oocytes, and can lead to luteinized unruputured follicle syndrome and corpus luteum defects.

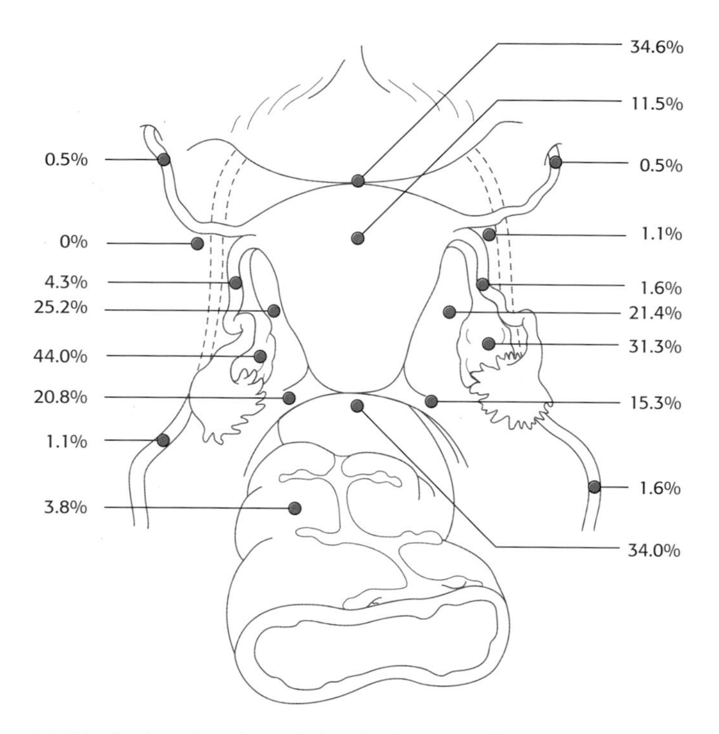

Figure 2.1 Distribution of endometriotic adhesions found at laparoscopy in 182 infertility patients. The figures represent the proportion of all patients with implants at that site. Reproduced with permission from Jenkins S *et al. Obstet Gynecol* 1986;67:335–8.

Macrophages. The number of macrophages in the peritoneal fluid is increased in women with pelvic endometriosis. This is associated with increased production of free radicals, which reduces sperm motility.

Ovulation disorders

Anovulation has been reported in 17–27% of patients with endometriosis. In some cases, combining treatment of the disease with ovulation induction increases the pregnancy rate.

Hyperprolactinaemia has been reported in several studies of patients with different stages of endometriosis. It seems, however, that the conditions co-exist and there is insufficient evidence to demonstrate a cause and effect relationship.

Abnormal follicular dynamics have been reported (i.e. abnormal rates of follicular development and premature follicular rupture).

Luteal phase defect, detected by out-of-phase endometrial development or asynchronous development of endometrial glands and stroma, could be the consequence of abnormal follicular development, inadequate production of progesterone, or lack of response of the endometrium to progesterone.

Luteinized unruptured follicle syndrome has been described in monkeys with surgically induced periovarian endometriosis. Theoretically, a decrease in the number of luteinizing hormone (LH) receptors could be the underlying mechanism, but ultrasound studies have failed to show a consistent increase in incidence of this syndrome in patients with endometriosis.

Pelvic pain

This can lead to a reduction in the frequency of intercourse and, therefore, reduce the likelihood of pregnancy.

Immunological abnormalities

T cells. As endometriosis involves transplantation of autologous endometrium and T cells are concerned with the rejection of homografts, changes in T-cell function have long been suspected in endometriosis. Controversy exists, however, regarding the pattern of circulating leukocytes, as some, but not all, investigators have reported decreased numbers of lymphocytes. To add confusion, increased numbers of T cells and B cells, and higher CD4:CD8 ratios in blood and peritoneal fluid have also been reported in women with endometriosis.

TABLE 2.2

Clinical pelvic factors and infertility in patients with moderate-to-severe endometriosis

- Adhesions distorting pelvic architecture, which interferes with oocyte releases and tubal pick-up
- Fimbrial distortion or occlusion
- Tubal narrowing and constriction
- Proximal tubal obstruction

Antigen-specific B-cell activation. Some researchers suggest that a subset of T cells is functionally deficient in women with endometriosis. Recently, a specific deficiency in lymphocyte-mediated cytotoxicity towards autologous endometrial cells was observed and was thought to be a result of natural killer (NK) cell dysfunction. The lowered cytotoxic effect has been confirmed by other investigators, but not the NK cell dysfunction. A definitive mechanism by which altered T-cell function could cause infertility has not yet emerged.

Anti-endometrial antibodies. Antibodies directed towards endometrial cell antigens have been reported in the serum of women with endometriosis, but why they exist is controversial. Anti-endometrial antibodies have also been detected in women with a wide range of pelvic pathology.

Non-specific B-cell activation. An autoimmune syndrome characterized by polyclonal B-cell activation has been suggested as a cause of infertility, though the exact mechanism is unclear.

Spontaneous abortion

An increased incidence of spontaneous abortion has been reported in patients with endometriosis, with a corresponding decrease after endometriosis has been treated. Abnormalities in prostaglandin function could be the possible mechanism. In a non-randomized study of patients with endometriosis, two-thirds of whom had suffered a previous miscarriage, the pregnancy rate was similar whether these patients had corrective surgery or not, but the miscarriage rate was higher in the group that had not been treated.

Implantation

Integrins are a group of compounds essential for cell adhesion. A deficiency of integrin av 3, a component of the embryo implantation cascade in the uterus, leads to a possible reduction in embryo implantation in women with early-stage endometriosis. However, this appears to be correctable when the disease is treated. This interesting theory awaits further investigation and clinical studies.

CHAPTER 3

Diagnosis

An accurate clinical assessment is essential to identify those women most at risk and those who require further evaluation (Table 3.1). Correct diagnosis will prevent unnecessary treatments, debilitating chronic pain and perhaps in younger sufferers, infertility.

Endometriosis is almost always detected during the reproductive years, most commonly between 25 and 29 years. The disease may also be found in early adolescents, especially those with Müllerian anomalies causing partial or complete obstruction, such as cervical atresia or obstructed rudimentary uterine horns. After the menopause, symptomatic endometriosis is typically associated with HRT.

A detailed history, including an association with any risk factors, is important. It is essential to ask about the family history, because growing evidence suggests that the disease has a genetic component. In patients with a family link, endometriosis tends to be at a more advanced stage and behaves in a more aggressive fashion at presentation.

Symptoms and signs

The most common symptoms of endometriosis are dysmenorrhoea and chronic pelvic pain unrelieved by analgesics (Table 3.2). Over half of affected patients complain of unilateral or bilateral pain, typically beginning 1–2 days before menstruation and lasting throughout the flow. Rectal pressure and low backache are also common symptoms.

The severity of pain does not correlate with the stage of the disease. Patients with minimal or mild endometriosis may have active disease and significant symptoms, while patients with severe endometriosis could be completely pain free. Over 50% of women with both pelvic pain and dysmenorrhoea are found to have endometriosis at laparoscopy.

The depth of infiltration of endometriosis in the uterosacral ligaments and the rectovaginal septum is positively associated with pelvic pain and dyspareunia. Many of these women also complain of pain during bowel motion while menstruating (dyschezia). Pain in the iliac fossae and flank may indicate involvement of the ureters, which may result in haematuria

TABLE 3.1

Diagnosis of endometriosis

History

- Reproductive age
- Short menstrual cycle (< 27 days)
- Partial or complete obstruction due to Müllerian anomalies
- Infertility or long gap since last pregnancy
- Family history of endometriosis

Symptoms and signs

- Chronic pelvic pain
- Dysmenorrhoea
- Dyspareunia
- Dyschezia
- Premenstrual spotting
- Menstrual irregularities
- Low back pain
- Gastrointestinal complaints
- Infertility

Physical findings

- Nodules along the uterosacral ligaments
- Adnexal masses due to endometriomas (e.g. ovarian cysts)
- Fixed retroversion of the uterus

Investigations

- Laparoscopy (the most useful diagnostic tool)
- Ultrasonography (endometriomas)
- MRI (endometriomas, adhesions, masses)
- Immunoassays (follow-up to therapy)

TABLE 3.2

Common symptoms of endometriosis*

Symptom	Incidence (%)
Dysmenorrhoea	60–80
Pelvic pain	30–50
Infertility	30–40
Dyspareunia	25–40
Menstrual irregularities	10–20
Cyclical dysuria/haematuria	1–2
Dyschezia (cyclic)	1–2
Rectal bleeding (cyclic)	< 1

* Reproduced with permission from Shaw RW. *An Atlas of Endometriosis*. Carnforth: Parthenon Publishing Group Ltd, 1993

and dysuria. Rectal bleeding occurs in about 20% of patients who have significant bowel endometriosis. Very occasionally, if an endometrioma is ruptured or bleeds, acute abdominal pain is the presenting symptom. The disease may be found in abdominal scars from previous surgery (e.g. Caesarean section) causing superficial cyclic pain, tenderness and swelling (Figure 3.1).

All types of abnormal bleeding, from premenstrual spotting to oligomenorrhea and hypermenorrhea, have been reported in patients.

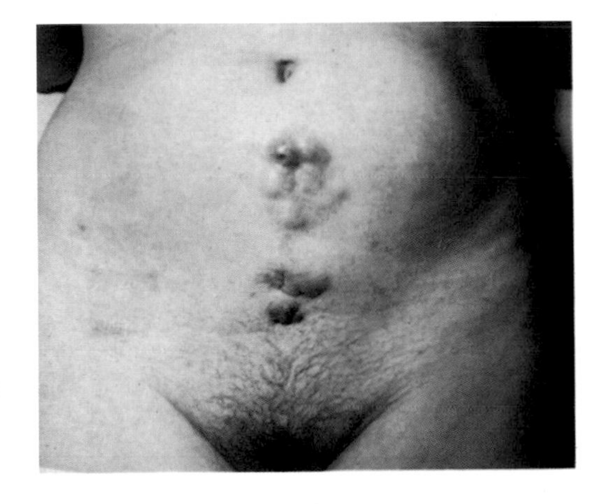

Figure 3.1 Endometriosis of an abdominal scar in a woman of 49 with a long history of the disease. Within 6 years it changed from being benign to being malignant. Reproduced with permission from Jeffcoate N. *Principles of Gynaecology*, 4th edition. London: Butterworth-Heinemann, 1975.

Physical examination

Pelvic endometriosis should be suspected if any of the following specific or non-specific findings are encountered during pelvic examination:

- multiple nodules along the uterosacral ligaments
- adnexal masses that may represent endometriomas
- rectovaginal endometriosis, which may be palpated by combined rectal and vaginal examination
- retroversion of the uterus, especially when it is fixed in position
- tenderness in the cul-de-sac in the absence of palpable pathology.

Differential diagnosis

It is important to be aware of the clinical diagnoses that endometriosis can mimic (Table 3.3). For example, endometriosis is commonly misdiagnosed as pelvic inflammatory disease (PID), and the true diagnosis is made only after several repeated courses of antibiotics and laparoscopy. Endometriosis is also occasionally diagnosed as acute appendicitis.

TABLE 3.3

Differential diagnosis

Differential diagnosis of endometriosis and acute pelvic pain

- Pelvic inflammatory disease (PID)
- Acute appendicitis
- Ovarian cysts (ruptured, torsion or infected)
- Ectopic pregnancy

Differential diagnosis of endometriosis and chronic pelvic pain

- Chronic pelvic inflammatory disease
- Adhesions as a result of previous surgery or infection
- Pelvic congestion syndrome
- Intermittent torsion of ovarian cyst
- Colitis and diverticulitis
- Chronic lumbosacral pain

Investigation and evaluation

Laparoscopy is the most important method of evaluating the pelvis, and should be considered the gold standard when endometriosis is suspected (Table 3.4). The accuracy of the diagnosis is dependent upon the skill of the laparoscopist and the thoroughness of the examination (microlaparoscopy may prove very useful for diagnosis in the near future). If spots of endometriosis are found they can be treated at the same time (Figure 3.2). The treatment or management that follows depends on the age and circumstances of the patient (see Chapter 4).

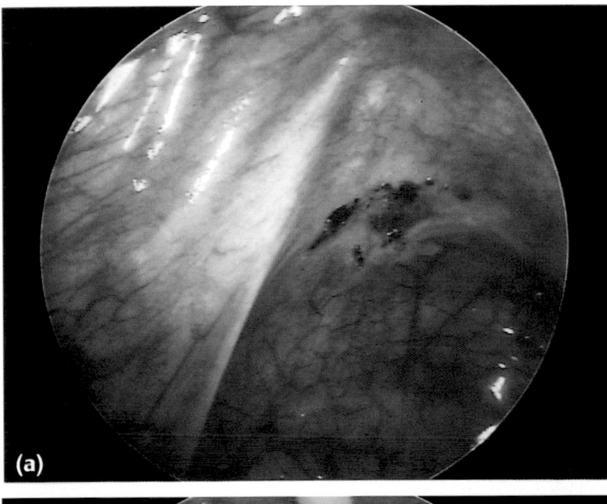

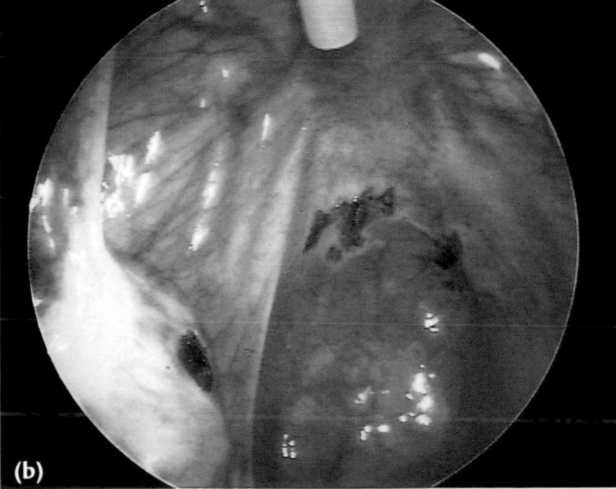

Figure 3.2 Laparoscopic appearance of lesion (a) before, and (b) after laser treatment.

TABLE 3.4

Laparoscopic examination

- Systematic and thorough evaluation of the pelvis
- Use second puncture probes and other instruments routinely
- Aspirate all peritoneal fluid
- Lyse adhesions
- Mobilize ovaries from the pelvic side wall
- Use rectal and vaginal probes
- Record the location, appearance and extent of the disease
- Video record the procedure routinely
- Thoroughly examine all atypical lesions (e.g. white nodules, translucent blebs, those with red flame-like appearance)

Imaging techniques. Selective use of imaging techniques, such as ultrasonography and MRI, can help to establish the extent of disease so that treatment can be planned. Other techniques (e.g. plain radiography and CT scanning) usually yield non-specific findings, but may be useful if endometriosis is suspected in the pleura or the bowel.

Ultrasonography should be performed using the transvaginal approach. The reliability of ultrasound depends on the nature of the lesions. In the detection of endometriomas, ultrasound is reported to have a sensitivity of 80% and specificity of 95%. In contrast, the sensitivity of ultrasound in the detection of focal implants is poor and may be as low as 10%. Typically, endometriomas are visualized as predominantly cystic masses with thick walls, often with diffuse acoustic enhancement or scattered internal echoes (Figure 3.3). Occasionally, endometriomas may contain septae, dependent echoes or fluid levels.

The diagnostic accuracy of ultrasound may be enhanced by Doppler flow studies. A scoring system that includes clinical parameters, CA-125 (see page 34), ultrasound and colour Doppler flow results has outstanding reliability, with both sensitivity and specificity above 99%.

MRI detects endometriomas, ovarian adhesions and extraperitoneal masses (Figure 3.4). It may be useful for noting changes in the size and number of endometriotic lesions during therapy, detecting invasion of nerves

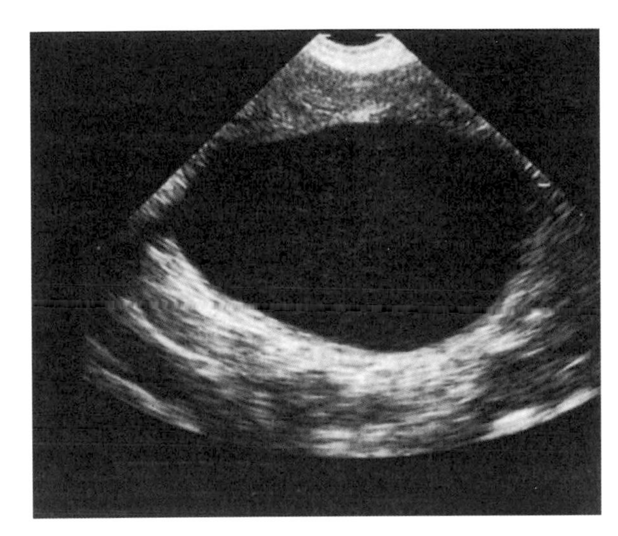

Figure 3.3 Ultrasound scan of an ovarian endometrioma with 'ground glass' appearance.

as in sciatic endometriosis, and for identifying abdominal wall lesions. MRI findings do not correlate with the stage of the disease.

Identification of endometriosis by MRI relies on the interpretation of pigmented haemorrhagic lesions. The signal characteristics vary according to the age of haemorrhage. Typically, the lesion appears hyperintense on T1-weighted images and hypointense on T2-weighted images (due to the presence of deoxyhaemoglobin and methaemoglobin). Identification of small implants may be better achieved with T1-weighted fat-suppressed images rather than with standard T1- and T2-weighted images. Addition of

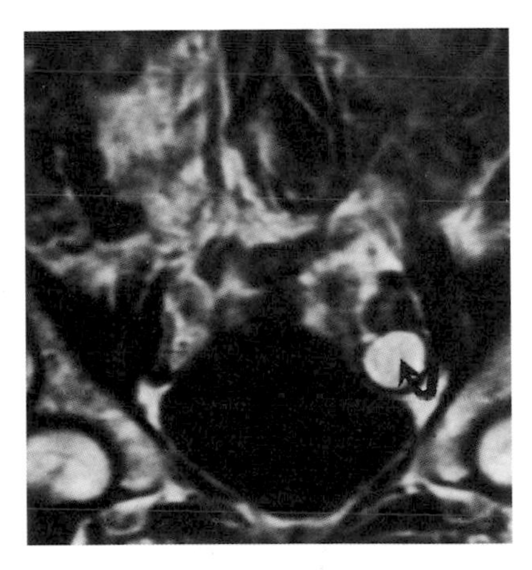

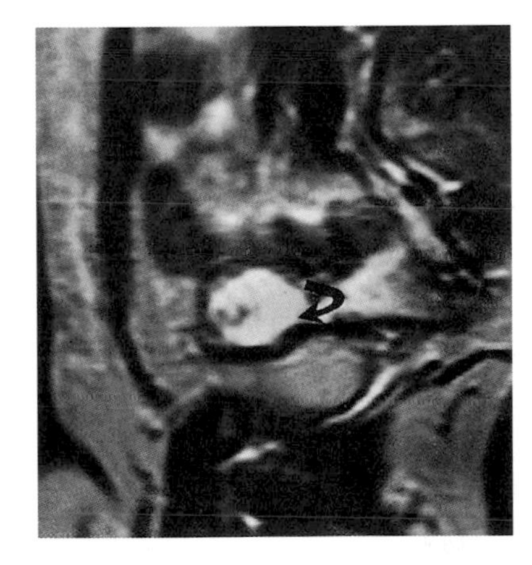

Figure 3.4 Endometrioma of the left ovary seen on MRI.

gadolinium-enhanced imaging has not been useful in providing further diagnostic information.

Immunoassays. Three serum immunoassays have been tried in the diagnosis of endometriosis: CA-125, placental protein 14 (PP14) and antibodies to endometrium. Of these, CA-125 shows the most promise.

CA-125 is an ovarian epithelial tumour antigen that is detected by a monoclonal antibody designated OC-125. The incidence of elevated CA-125 levels increases with the severity of the disease and mean concentrations correlate clearly with disease stage. However, because CA-125 levels are not elevated in mild forms of endometriosis, and are elevated during and immediately after menstruation, CA-125 is not useful as a screening test. It could, however, be valuable in monitoring the effects of therapy. CA-125 measurement has been successfully used in conjunction with other examinations (e.g. ultrasonography).

CHAPTER 4

Medical treatment

A young woman aged between 16 and 20 years, who has severe period pain and does not respond to analgesics, should have laparoscopy to confirm the diagnosis before medical treatment is given. This is preventive medicine – because the disease is progressive, it may cause a massive distortion of the pelvis, which could affect fertility later. If infertility is the problem, laparoscopy should be performed as soon as possible so assisted conception can begin (Chapter 6).

Hormonal therapy

This has been the main medical treatment for endometriosis for half a century. In the 1940s and 1950s, diethylstilbestrol and methyltestosterone were used, but were abandoned because the side-effects were too great. In the 1960s, progestogen alone or combined oestrogen/progestogen preparations were used in an attempt to produce a pseudopregnancy state (see below), but again significant side-effects caused their decline. Danazol was introduced in the early 1970s, and led to the use of gonadotrophin-releasing hormone (GnRH) agonists in the next decade. More recently, GnRH antagonists and anti-progesterones have been used with favourable reports.

Pseudopregnancy. In 1959, Kistner reported the use of Enovid (norethynodrel and mestranol) in 58 women with pelvic endometriosis. It was a landmark in the history of pharmacological treatment of endometriosis, but it lost popularity because of both oestrogenic and progestational side-effects.

Danazol is a synthetic by-product of testosterone, with a half life of 4.5 hours. Peak levels are reached 2 hours after oral ingestion and it is undetectable after 8 hours. It is metabolized in the liver, and the principle metabolite, methylethisterone, exhibits mild progestrogenic and androgenic activity.

Danazol has a direct effect on steroidogenesis, acting on cholesterol cleavage enzymes, and on intracellular steroid receptors. It has an indirect

TABLE 4.1

Progestogens used in the treatment of endometriosis

Progestogens alone
• Oral medroxyprogesterone acetate
• Injectable medroxyprogesterone acetate
• Norethisterone/norethindrone
• Megestrol acetate
• Dydrogesterone
Progestogens in combination with oestrogens
• Desogestrel
• Cyproterone acetate

action by decreasing GnRH pulse frequency, which may suppress ovulation.

Side-effects. The most common are related to the hyperandrogenic state – weight gain, oily skin and hair, nausea, acne, muscle cramps and hirsutism. Deepening of the voice, though uncommon, is irreversible. Hypo-oestrogenic side-effects, such as hot flushes, decreased breast size and reduced libido may also occur.

Danazol has multiple metabolic side-effects, the most important of which relate to blood cholesterol. It decreases HDL and increases LDL levels, which must be taken into account as the drug is given for long periods (6–9 months). Its use should be avoided in women with a history of liver disease. During treatment with danazol, women should be advised to use barrier methods of contraception, such as condoms.

Gestrinone is a progesterone agonist/antagonist that has been used in Europe for treatment of endometriosis, but is unavailable in the USA at the time of press. The actions of gestrinone result in amenorrhea and endometrial atrophy, similar to other androgen steroid analogues (e.g. danazol). It acts both centrally and peripherally to reduce oestradiol and obliterate the mid-cycle luteinizing hormone (LH) surge.

Gestrinone has a long half-life allowing oral administration 2–3 times weekly. In randomized clinical trials, gestrinone was effective in reducing the painful symptoms of endometriosis.

Side-effects. Gestrinone has fewer androgenic symptomatic and metabolic effects compared with danazol, and fewer hypo-oestrogenic side-effects. During treatment with gestrinone, women should be advised to use barrier methods of contraception, such as condoms.

Progestogens. The effect of progestogens (synthetic progesterone preparations) on endometrial tissue depends on the dosage, length of treatment and the activity of the individual progestogen (Table 1.1).

Side-effects include irregular vaginal bleeding, weight gain, fluid retention, breast tenderness and mood changes.

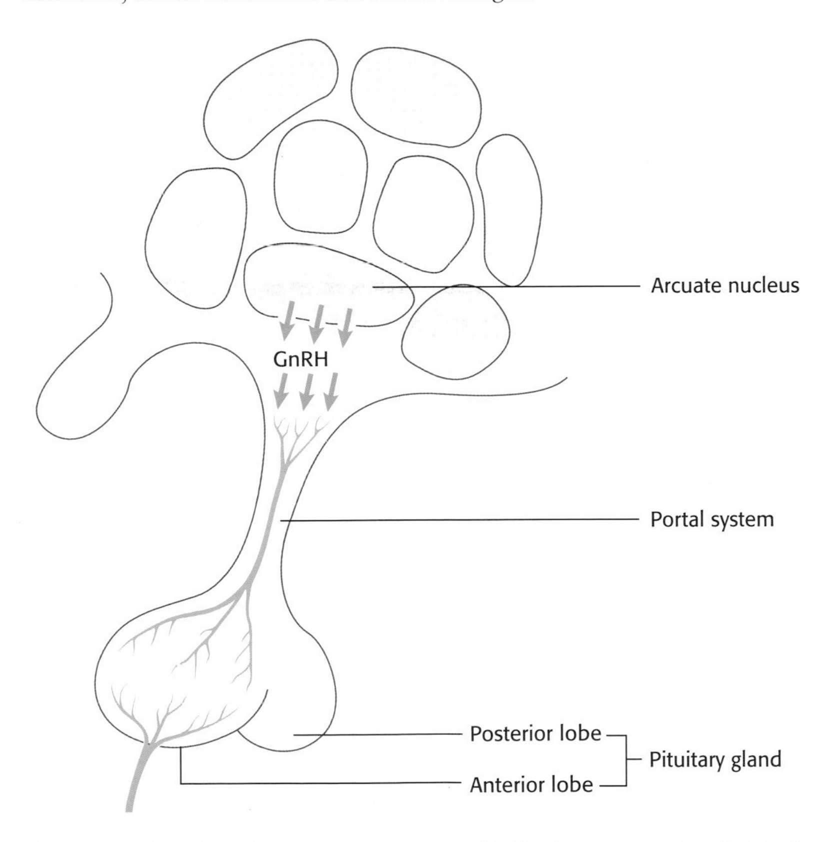

Figure 4.1 Gonadotrophin-releasing hormone (GnRH) is secreted primarily into the portal circulation by the arcuate nucleus. It is then carried to the gonadotrope cell in the anterior pituitary, where it stimulates the synthesis, storage and release of luteinizing hormone (LH) and follicle-stimulating hormone (FSH).

GnRH agonists. Native GnRH is a short-acting decapeptide that is secreted episodically into the pituitary circulation to regulate the release of LH and follicle-stimulating hormone (FSH). Continuous exposure to GnRH leads to down-regulation of pituitary function, which suppresses ovarian steroid production inducing a reversible pseudomenopause (Figure 4.1). Long-acting agonist analogues of GnRH capitalize on these effects. The medications must be given parenterally and are available as a nasal spray (nafarelin, buserelin), subcutaneous pellet (goserelin) or depot injection (leuprolide; Table 4.2). All these medications help to reduce pain associated with endometriosis.

Side-effects. The side-effects of the GnRH agonists are similar to those caused by lack of oestrogen. Bone loss may occur and bones may take 6–12 months to recover when treatment is completed.

GnRH agonist add-back therapy. Patients at high risk of osteoporosis can be given oestrogen/progestogen HRT to counter the adverse impact of prolonged hypo-oestrogenism. GnRH agonists can be used with add-back therapy in various regimens (Figure 4.2). Those of proven efficacy in the treatment of endometriosis include progestogen alone, progestogen and oestrogen combinations, or progestogen bisphosphonates.

Both the 17-hydroxyprogesterone derivative, medroxyprogesterone acetate, and 19-nortestosterone derivative, norethisterone (UK)/norethindrone (USA), have an established ability to promote

TABLE 4.2

Reduction in pain scores after treatment with a GnRH analogue*

	Depot leuprolide injection		Placebo		Significance
	n	Mean change in pain score	n	Mean change in pain score	
Dysmenorrhoea	28	+2.2	21	−0.2	$p < 0.001$
Pelvic pain	28	−1.2	21	−0.3	$p = 0.001$
Dyspareunia	17	−0.4	13	0.1	ns
Pelvic tenderness	28	+1.0	21	−0.3	$p = 0.001$

* Dlugi *et al.* 1990

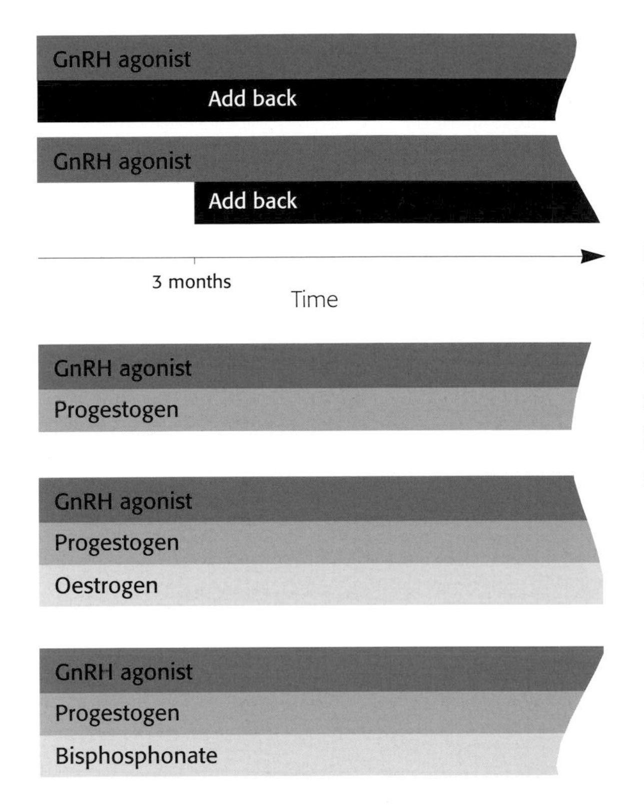

Figure 4.2 Options for gonadotrophin-releasing hormone (GnRH) add-back regimens, to protect bones while the disease is treated.

endometrial atrophy (pseudopregnancy). In this sense, the addition of progestogen only to a long-term GnRH regimen provides a multi-modal attack on the pathophysiology of endometriosis.

In terms of the impact on bone density, progestogen-only add-back therapy is sufficient to eliminate the GnRH-induced decrease in radial bone density (as shown by single-photon absorptiometry). Similarly, combinations of nafarelin and norethisterone/norethindrone or histrelin and medroxyprogesterone acetate prove protective of the lumbar spine (as shown by dual-photon absorptiometry). In contrast, treatment with histrelin and norethisterone/norethindrone do not protect from GnRH induced decrease in lumbar bone density. The use of depot leuprolide in conjunction with norethisterone/norethindrone, 5–10 mg daily, is associated with a decrease in lumbar bone density of 2.7% after 6 months' therapy. Both norethisterone/norethindrone and medroxyprogesterone acetate combat the symptom of hot flushes.

Antiprogesterones. Mifepristone, known as RU-486, has been used for pregnancy termination and other medical indications. It has been shown to inhibit ovulation and disrupt endometrial integrity, and has been used in trials in patients with symptomatic endometriosis to induce chronic anovulation.

In two pilot studies, RU-486, 100 mg/day, was given for 3 months with significant improvement in pelvic pain, though there was no visible regression of endometriosis; in a follow-up study, treatment was extended to 6 months and the dose lowered to 50 mg/day, causing a significant decrease in pelvic pain within 4 weeks.

These pilot studies indicate a potential role for antiprogesterones in the treatment of endometriosis. More than 400 different antiprogesterone analogues have been synthesized worldwide and they may have a realistic place in the future treatment of the disease.

Nonsteroidal anti-inflammatory drugs are useful in the treatment of painful menstruation associated with endometriosis. Ibuprofen and naproxen have been found to improve symptoms significantly.

CHAPTER 5

Surgical treatment

Surgery is used for the diagnosis and treatment of endometriosis. The choice of procedure depends on the stage of endometriosis, the site of the disease and whether the patient wants to have a child. The objectives of surgery are to:

- relieve symptoms
- restore fertility
- remove endometriotic implants
- delay recurrence of the disease.

Laparoscopic surgery

The major advantage of laparoscopy is that it allows diagnostic as well as therapeutic procedures (Table 5.1) to be performed at the same time, with minimal and gentle manipulation of tissues to avoid trauma. If endometriosis is found, it should be ablated or removed, preferably using laser surgery to reduce tissue damage. It is also possible to combine assisted conception techniques with treatment of the disease.

The principles of laparoscopic surgery for endometriosis are:

- eradication of all visible disease by removal, vaporization or destruction

TABLE 5.1

Laparoscopic procedures for treatment of endometriosis

- Adhesiolysis
- Removal of ovarian endometriomas
- Oophorectomy
- Resection of bladder endometriosis
- Resection of ureteric endometriosis
- Resection of invasive bowel endometriosis
- Appendicectomy
- Laparoscopic-assisted vaginal hysterectomy
- Laparoscopic uterosacral nerve ablation
- Laparascopic presacral neurectomy

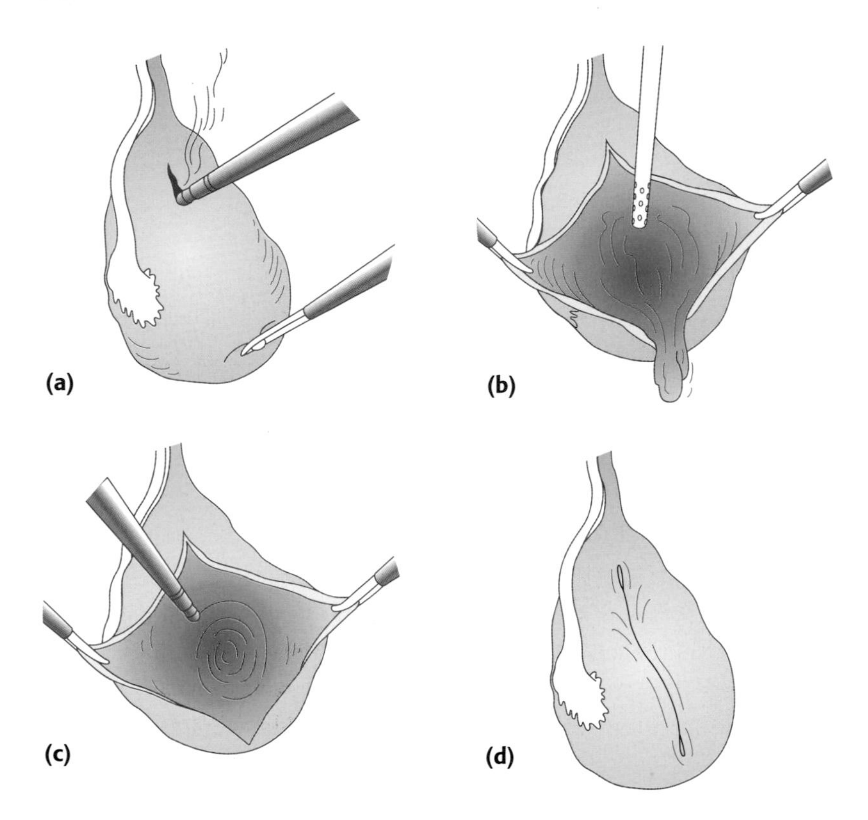

Figure 5.1 Laparoscopic treatment of ovarian endometriomas: (a) the ovary is grasped and the cyst is entered with a laser probe; (b) the cyst is washed out with the irrigator/aspirator so the cyst wall can be examined; (c) the laser probe destroys the cyst wall, starting from the bottom and moving towards the top in a spiral fashion; (d) the cyst edges fold towards each other with no need for suturing.

- biopsy of ovarian cystic lesions or suspicious areas before laser application
- thorough examination of the peritoneal cavity and ovarian lesions before the cyst is entered
- restoration of normal anatomy
- complete haemostasis.

Laparoscopy is indicated in women with:

- infertility of more than a year's duration
- pelvic pain unresponsive to medical treatment for 3–6 months
- adnexal masses that may indicate endometriomas.

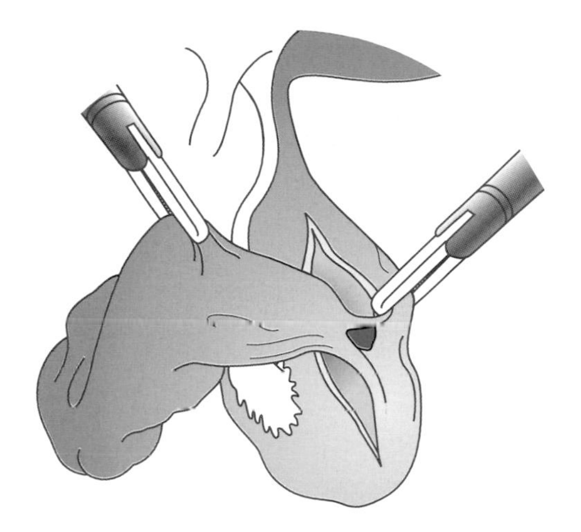

Figure 5.2 Laparoscopic view of the cyst wall being separated from the ovarian cortex.

Laparoscopic treatment of ovarian endometriomas. The cyst wall is opened laparoscopically and the chocolate fluid aspirated. As the wall is invariably adherent to the ovarian tissue, destruction of the wall is achieved by vaporization with laser, starting from the bottom and moving towards the top in a spiral fashion (Figure 5.1). Where the cyst is not adherent to the ovary, the cyst is stripped intact by hydrodissection or sharp dissection (Figure 5.2). Superficial and residual endometriotic spots should be treated using CO_2 laser ablation.

Second-look laparoscopy is an appropriate procedure in patients who have undergone laparoscopy for the resection of endometriosis or who have residual pain. It is usually scheduled 1–6 weeks after the initial surgery to check if any endometriotic spots were missed and allows separation of the *de novo* adhesions that are still relatively filmy in consistency. It also provides an opportunity to assess the prognosis for fertility.

Radical surgery

In the early days, surgical removal of the uterus was the sole treatment for endometriosis. Nowadays it is usually reserved for patients with intractable pain who have completed their family and for women in whom conservative surgery has failed. At least 12% of all endometriosis patients require radical surgery.

Definitive surgery offers prompt, complete and long-term relief of pain

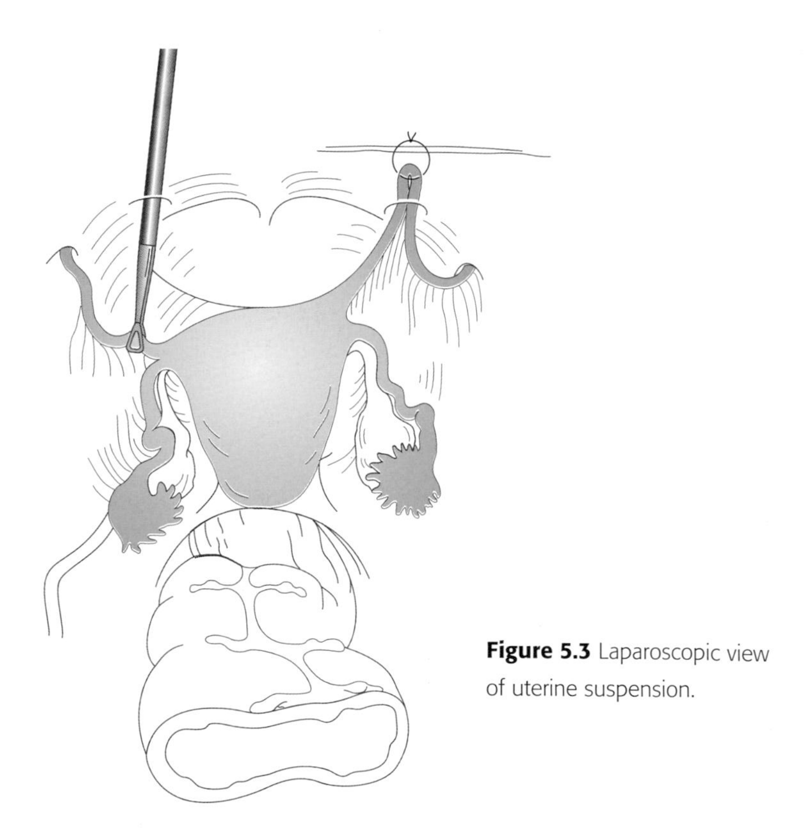

Figure 5.3 Laparoscopic view of uterine suspension.

compared with medical treatment. Most hysterectomies are performed by the abdominal route though, in selected cases, if laparoscopy reveals a free cul-de-sac or allows lysis of adhesions, then vaginal hysterectomy can be performed safely. When the posterior cul-de-sac is obliterated and extensive fibrosis is present deep in the pelvis, subtotal hysterectomy may be indicated.

The recurrence of cyclic pain associated with endometriosis after hysterectomy with preservation of normal ovaries is only about 3%.

HRT. The decision to perform curative radical surgery in a young woman is always very difficult but, if it is contemplated, HRT should be discussed and implemented both for the cardiovascular benefits as well as to prevent osteoporosis. Although the risk of recurrence of endometriosis as a result of HRT is negligible, it may be wise to add progestogen to oestrogen if the disease is incompletely resected or deeply invasive, if there are atypical changes or if symptoms recur.

Adjunctive procedures for pelvic pain

The surgical technique used to treat pelvic pain will depend on where the pain occurs.

Uterine suspension. This is usually performed to prevent recurrence of adhesions in the cul-de-sac and to minimize dyspareunia from central endometriosis. It corrects fixed retroversion of the uterus and allows better access of the Fallopian tubes to the Pouch of Douglas (Figure 5.3).

Laparoscopic uterosacral nerve ablation (LUNA). This procedure is likely to benefit patients with significant central dysmenorrhoea. It will not benefit those with lateral pelvic pain or pain of gastrointestinal or urinary tract origin. It also has no benefit in terms of treating infertility. It should not be performed if the anatomy of the ureters and cul-de-sac is unclear.

In controlled studies, the short-term success rate of LUNA in the relief of pain is 50–70%. Complications include haemorrhage, especially if the ablation is taken too far laterally or posteriorly.

Figure 5.4 Presacral neurectomy.

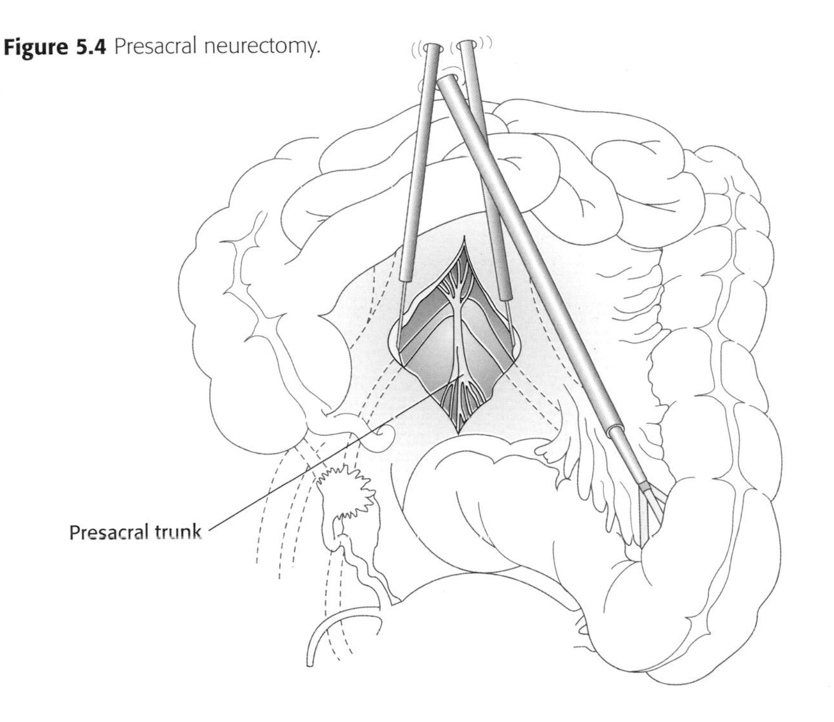

Presacral neurectomy. This procedure (Figure 5.4) is used to treat patients with midline pelvic pain. It can be performed conventionally or microsurgically. There is no evidence that the procedure enhances fertility or affects menstruation.

The presacral nerve is the superior hypogastric plexus that supplies efferent stimulation to the vessel. The most common immediate complication of presacral neurectomy is bleeding from the middle sacral artery or vein, or from the inferior mesenteric artery or its superior haemorrhoidal branch. Bleeding can usually be prevented by meticulous surgical technique.

Laparoscopic presacral neurectomy is accomplished using high-resolution laparoscopy and a video camera. Five puncture sites are usual with a fan retractor to move the rectosigmoid colon. The presacral nerve bundles are identified, dissected free and elevated.

A variety of techniques are used for excision, including endoloop suture ligation with excision of intervening nerve bundle, bipolar cauterization of the nerve bundles with resection of intervening segment, and a combination of bipolar cautery and Nd-Yag laser.

The main complications are bleeding and injury to the ureter, though other problems have been reported including urinary bladder dysfunction, constipation and vaginal dryness. The overall success of the procedure exceeds 50%.

CHAPTER 6

Treatment of associated infertility

Approaches to the treatment of infertility associated with endometriosis include:

- surgical
- medical
- expectant (i.e. no treatment)
- combined medical and surgical
- analgesic (NSAIDs).

Efficacy of surgical treatment

Surgical versus non-surgical approaches. The surgical approach (laparoscopy or laparotomy) is significantly superior to non-surgical treatment (no treatment or medical treatment) for all stages of endometriosis-associated infertility. A meta-analysis of data comparing surgical with non-surgical treatment showed the surgical approach increased pregnancy rates by 38%, and confidence intervals were 28–48% higher.

Surgical treatment of minimal and mild endometriosis. Expectant management has been the traditional approach, achieving an average pregnancy rate of approximately 45%, and a monthly fecundity of 6.8%. Surgical treatment produces a higher pregnancy rate. Maheux and colleagues from France reported a multicentre, prospective, double-blind, controlled, randomized study in which laparoscopic treatment resulted in a significantly higher pregnancy rate than expectant management 9 months after treatment (Figure 6.1).

Surgical treatment of moderate and severe endometriosis. Surgery is the treatment of choice in patients with moderate and severe endometriosis, as the associated anatomical distortion can be corrected at the same time.

Efficacy of medical treatment

There is solid evidence that medical therapy alone does not improve fertility potential. The data from randomized controlled studies have been

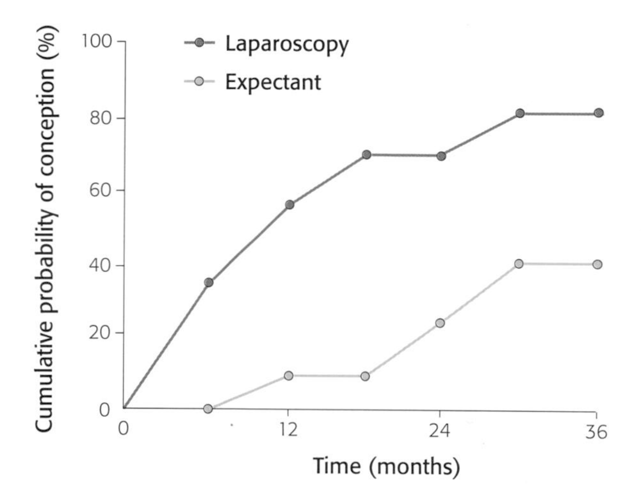

Figure 6.1 Conception rates in women with mild endometriosis treated laparoscopically or managed expectantly.

homogeneous despite different interventions and designs. The additional costs, side-effects and the need for requisite contraception render the medical option inadvisable in patients with endometriosis-associated infertility.

In contrast, medical therapy is very effective in reducing the pain associated with endometriosis. Generally, 80–90% of patients receiving GnRH agonists or other treatment will experience significant improvement in the disease, and recurrence rates correlate with the severity of the disease. The side-effect profile is the most important factor in choosing a particular medical therapy.

Expectant management

The biggest disadvantage of medical treatment for minimal endometriosis associated with infertility is that it induces anovulation for 6–9 months therefore preventing these women from becoming pregnant. Expectant management is adopted by many to good effect (Table 6.1).

Combined medical and surgical treatment

Malinak has observed a cyclicity in the popularity of medical versus surgical treatment of endometriosis over the years. It is common practice in the 1990s for the therapies to be used simultaneously to treat the disease.

Theoretically, pre-operative medical treatment should:

- facilitate surgical technique

- reduce pelvic vascularization and inflammation
- increase pregnancy success
- lower the risk of recurrence of the disease
- prevent delay between surgery and attempt at pregnancy.

Similarly, postoperative medical therapy should:

- cure residual disease following surgery
- not mask pre-operative treatment.

Currently, clinical data are insufficient to evaluate pre-operative treatment.

TABLE 6.1

Expectant management in patients with infertility and mild endometriosis

Study	n	Pregnancy (%)	Pregnancy rate (%/month)
Garcia and David 1977	17	64.7	5
Schenken and Malinak 1982	18	72.2	10.2
Siebel *et al.* 1982	28	14	11.1
Portuondo *et al.* 1983	31	61.2	8.3
Olive *et al.* 1985	34	52.9	5.7
Hull *et al.* 1987	56	37.5	
Bayer *et al.* 1988	36	47.2	
Total	**220**	**49.1%**	

Combined data from studies between 1984 and 1993 show that medical therapy after surgery is not better than laparoscopy or laparotomy alone. The homogeneity of the studies in this comparison strengthens the conclusion that no difference in outcome exists. Also, the costs, side-effects and delayed fertility argue against any role for medical therapy in the postoperative period.

Laparoscopy or laparotomy?

The laparoscopic approach has been popularized because of significant improvement in equipment and operative techniques. Adamson and colleagues carried out a life-table analysis of patients with minimal or mild endometriosis, but with no other infertility factors. They found similar outcomes between laparoscopy and laparotomy. For moderate or severe disease, laparoscopy had better pregnancy results than laparotomy. Their meta-analysis of the studies also observed no significant difference in pregnancy rates. Therefore, depending on the individual situation, the primary surgical approach should be laparoscopy, which offers the following advantages over laparotomy:

- better visualization
- less tissue trauma
- less adhesion formation
- shorter recovery time
- equivalent, if not better, success rates.

Ovarian endometriomas. Laparoscopic treatment resulted in pregnancy rates of 50% (26 of 52) and 52% (12 of 23) in two different studies of women with ovarian endometriomas. In a prospective cohort study comparing the two treatments, the estimated cumulative pregnancy rate at 3 years was 52% for laparoscopy and 42% for laparotomy (Figure 6.2). With improved techniques, laparoscopy has become the standard approach for drainage and excision of endometriomas, with these observations:

- recurrence rate is approximately 10%
- *de novo* adhesion formation is approximately 20%
- incidence of recurring adhesions is approximately 80%
- normal ovarian function is retained after conservative surgery.

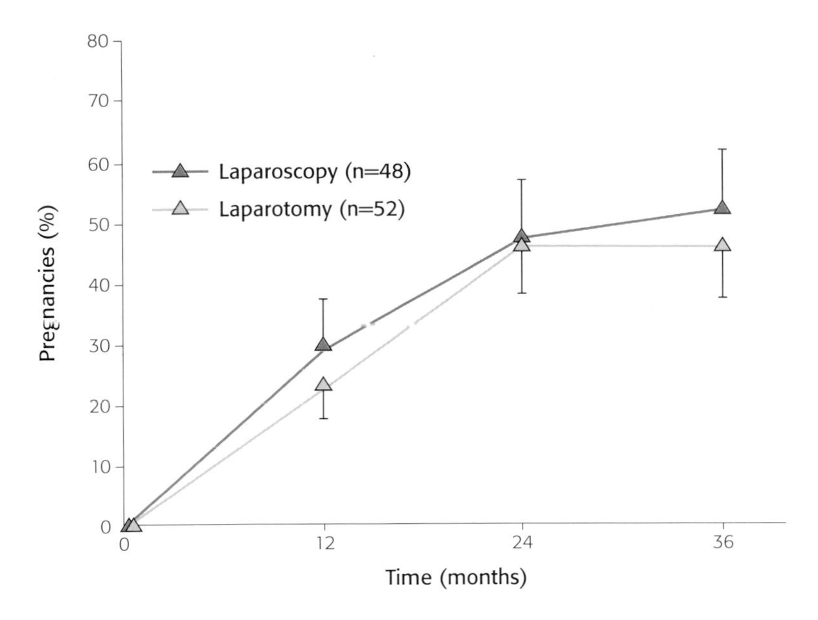

Figure 6.2 Estimated cumulative life-table pregnancy rates for laparoscopy versus laparotomy for the treatment of endometriomas. Reproduced with permission from Adamson GD *et al. Fertil Steril* 1992;57:965–73.

Endometriosis in the posterior cul-de-sac and rectovaginal septum. In a study by Reich and colleagues, laparoscopic surgery of partial or complete cul-de-sac obliteration resulted in a 74% pregnancy rate. However, over one-third of the patients required more than one laparoscopy. In another study by Adamson and colleagues, life-table pregnancy rates for patients with complete posterior cul-de-sac obliteration was 29.6% for those treated laparoscopically compared with 23.7% for those treated by laparotomy.

CHAPTER 7

Assisted reproductive technology and endometriosis

While medical treatment of endometriosis is successful in terms of relief of pain and symptoms, no control studies have shown its efficacy in improving the outcome of fertility treatment. For those patients with endometriosis who have undergone medical or surgical therapy, or both, assisted reproductive technology (ART) offers hope. Techniques include:

- controlled ovarian hyperstimulation (COH)
- intrauterine insemination (IUI)
- *in-vitro* fertilization (IVF)
- gamete intrafallopian transfer (GIFT)
- intracytoplasmic sperm injection (ICSI).

COH and IUI

Several studies have demonstrated the efficacy of COH and IUI. The advantages are substantial and include:

- increased number of oocytes available for fertilization
- higher levels of follicular and luteal phase gonadal steroids
- increased number of sperm present at the fertilization site
- optimized likelihood of gamete interaction between the oocytes and sperm.

The generally accepted fecundity of normal couples is about 20%. In patients with endometriosis or unexplained infertility, it varies from 1% to 3%, depending on the age of the female partner, whether a pregnancy has previously been achieved, and the duration of infertility. Haney and colleagues have shown that COH and IUI in women with endometriosis gives a cycle fecundity rate approaching the norm (Table 7.1), except in cases of severe endometriosis.

Results of studies

- Human menopausal gonadotrophins (hMG) and IUI versus hMG and intercourse – monthly fecundity rate (MFR) in the IUI group was 13%, while that in the intercourse group was 7%.
- COH and IUI cycles versus expectant management – MFR in the COH

TABLE 7.1

COH and IUI in women with endometriosis

Stage of endometriosis	Cycle fecundity (%)
Minimal	16
Mild	10
Moderate	18
Severe	0
Total	**14**

and IUI group was 15%, while that in the expectant group was 5%; cumulative pregnancy rates were 37% and 24%, respectively.

- Superovulation–intrauterine insemination (SO–IUI) gave a clinical pregnancy rate of 20.5%/patient; 96% of the pregnancies occurred in the first two cycles.
- Patients in an hMG IUI treatment group demonstrated a constant fecundity rate until after 40 years of age. At 12 months after surgery, 57% under 35 years and 33% over 35 years had conceived. By 24 months, 77% of patients under 35 years had conceived, while 39% of those aged 35 years or more had conceived. When hMG IUI was initiated 6 months after surgery in women over 35 years, 81% achieved pregnancy within 16 months of surgery. In contrast, when hMG IUI was started 12 months after surgery in women under 35 years, 88% achieved pregnancy compared with 77% not treated with hMG IUI.

Conclusions. hMG IUI improves infertility associated with endometriosis, taking into account surgery, age and stage of disease. Women aged 35 years or over, and women with moderate and severe disease, appear to benefit most from hMG IUI soon after surgery. Superovulation is an effective treatment for patients with endometriosis who have patent Fallopian tubes.

IVF

Recent results published by the Human Fertilization and Embryology Authority (HFEA) in the UK, the French National Registry and those of the US Society of Reproductive Technology (SART) show no significant difference between IVF and embryo transfer (ET) in achieving pregnancy in patients with endometriosis and other indications associated with infertility. Pregnancy and birth rates achieved with IVF in women with different causes of infertility are shown in Table 7.2. The pregnancy rate achieved with IVF in women with endometriosis decreases with age (Figure 7.1).

Conclusions. IVF is an effective alternative to re-operation, particularly if initial surgery failed to restore fertility. Women with mild or moderate endometriosis might be advised to go directly to IVF. In more severe cases, it is advisable to operate to reduce or remove the disease before starting IVF treatment.

TABLE 7.2

IVF clinical pregnancy and live birth rates for female causes of infertility*

Factor	Clinical pregnancy rate (%)	Live birth rate (%)
Tubal disease	16.9	13.3
Endometriosis	18.6	15.0
Unexplained	19.0	15.9

* Data from Human Fertilization and Embryology Authority, 6th Annual Report.

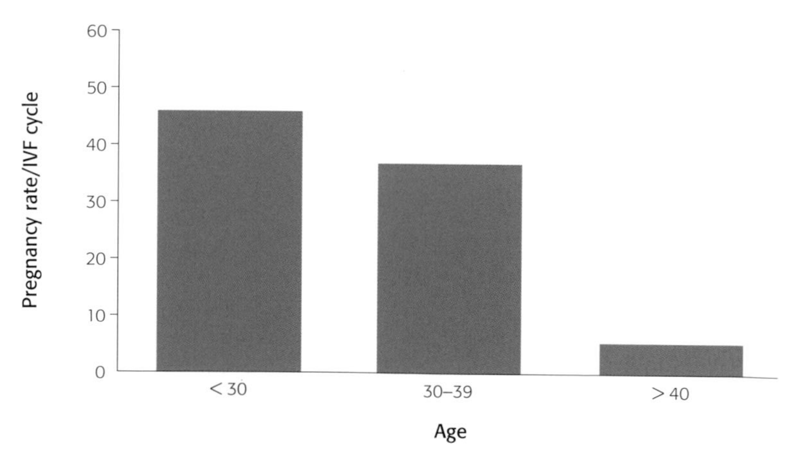

Figure 7.1 Pregnancy rate per IVF cycle in patients with endometriosis related to age (Lister Hospital, UK, 1988–1996).

GIFT

GIFT has been associated with a high pregnancy rate in women with endometriosis. When GIFT and laser treatment for the disease are combined, studies show even greater success rates; for example, 45%/65% pregnancy rates compared with 36%/34% in women not receiving concurrent treatment. The pregnancy rate was increased to 55% in women with minimal and mild endometriosis when a short course of GnRH agonist was given before hMG stimulation.

ICSI

ICSI has become the most widely applied method of assisted fertilization for male infertility. A retrospective study has assessed the impact of endometriosis on the outcome of ICSI. There was a significant reduction in the number of oocytes retrieved from women with endometriosis compared with those without, but there were no significant differences in either fertilization or pregnancy and implantation rates.

CHAPTER 8

Extrapelvic endometriosis

Extrapelvic endometriosis is estimated to occur in between 1% and 10% of patients with pelvic endometriosis. The disease has been reported to occur in almost all body structures, but the most common sites are the intestine, urinary tract, distal areas in the abdominal cavity, extrapelvic genital structures, lungs, skin and nervous system.

Gastrointestinal tract

Up to 50% of women with severe endometriosis have gastrointestinal endometriosis, the most common sites being the rectosigmoid colon (50%), appendix (15%), small bowel (14%), rectum (14%), and the caecum and colon (5%) (Figure 8.1). The symptoms of gastrointestinal endometriosis are listed in Table 8.1.

Endometriosis of the appendix may present as an incidental finding with or without pelvic disease. The appendix should be inspected in all patients undergoing surgery for endometriosis, as should the Meckel's diverticulum; if the disease is found, it should be removed.

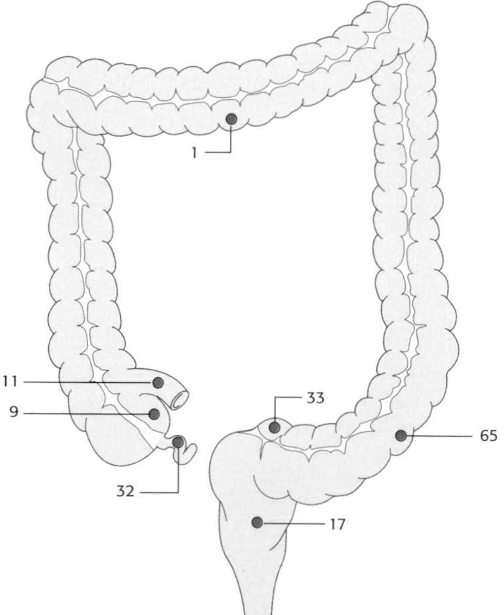

Figure 8.1 Sites of 168 lesions in 163 patients with endometriosis of the bowel. Data from Weed JC *et al. Obstet Gynecol* 1987;69:727–30.

TABLE 8.1

Symptoms of gastrointestinal endometriosis

- Diarrhoea
- Constipation
- Perimenstrual changes in bowel habits
- Rectal bleeding
- Pain with defecation
- Tenesmus
- Abdominal distension
- Small stools
- Colicky abdominal pain

Urinary tract

Urinary tract endometriosis is thought to affect 1–4% of women with pelvic endometriosis; there have also been many cases without pre or postoperative evidence of pelvic disease. Ureteral obstruction is associated with major morbidity; up to 30% of patients suffer loss of kidney function, though renal endometriosis itself is extremely rare.

The bladder is the most common site of endometriosis in the urinary tract (80–90% of cases), usually occurring in the trigone, dorsal wall, at the uterovesicular junction or transmurally. The ureters are involved in 10–15% of cases, with the left being more commonly affected than the right; urethral lesions are usually found in the distal third of the ureter below the pelvic brim.

The symptoms of urinary tract endometriosis are listed in Table 8.2. The diagnosis can be confirmed by:

- ultrasound
- CT and MRI
- cystoscopy
- biopsy – also used to exclude malignancy.

In most cases, however, ureteral and renal involvement are diagnosed at the time of open surgical procedure.

Treatment decisions should be based on renal function, the extent and location of the disease, severity of symptoms, age of patient and desire for

TABLE 8.2

Symptoms of urinary tract endometriosis

- Dysuria
- Frequency
- Superpubic pressure
- Back pain

future pregnancy. If renal function is near normal, hormonal therapy can generally be attempted. Surgery is required for ureteral involvement if there is significant fibrosis and the disease does not respond to hormone treatment.

The recurrence rate of endometriosis in the bladder and ureters is usually very high after medication is stopped, so duration of therapy is important.

Surgery is indicated in cases of acute urinary tract obstruction or when symptoms are severe despite hormonal therapy. The primary surgical treatment of renal endometriosis has been nephrectomy. In patients with bladder endometriosis, partial cystectomy can be performed with good long-term outcome (Figure 8.2).

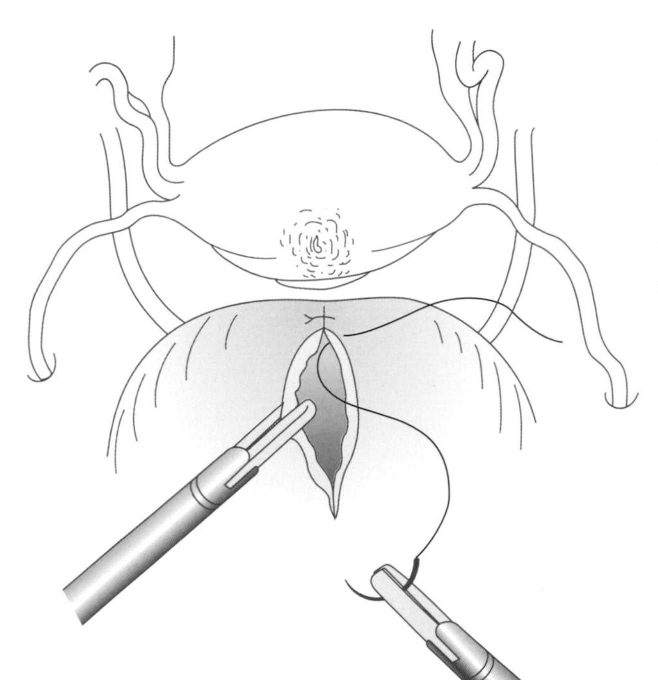

Figure 8.2 Partial cystectomy for the treatment of bladder endometriosis. The bladder wall is repaired in one layer.

Thorax

Just over 100 cases of thoracic endometriosis have been reported in the USA and UK. The disease appears to affect women slightly older than those with pelvic endometriosis, with an average age of 35 years. Between 50% and 80% of patients have co-existing pelvic endometriosis.

The most common presenting symptom is pneumothorax, followed by haemothorax, haemoptysis and asymptomatic lung nodule. Pleural lesions are more likely to cause pneumothorax or haemothorax; haemoptysis is generally the result of lesions in the lung parenchyma.

Total abdominal hysterectomy with bilateral salpingo-oophorectomy has been used in the past as the main treatment for extirpation of the origin of thoracic endometriosis. More recently, GnRH agonists and danazol have been used with success in several case reports.

Diaphragm

Diaphragmatic endometriosis may present as pain in the right upper quadrant or referred pain in the right shoulder. An increasing number of cases have been reported. In one case, a pregnant patient developed haemoperitoneum because of bleeding from an ectopic fetus that had implanted on diaphragmatic endometriosis.

Implantation of viable endometrial cells probably occurs following circulation of the cells in a clockwise fashion in the peritoneal fluid. The usual treatment – GnRH agonists and surgery – is reserved for patients with acute symptoms or those who do not respond to other measures. Laparoscopic treatment has also been reported.

Cutaneous endometriosis

Endometriosis involving the skin is limited to the anterior abdominal wall at or below the umbilicus.

Umbilical endometriosis classically presents as a bluish, tender mass, often associated with bleeding. The lesions can be evaluated radiographically or by ultrasound, but the best method is excision biopsy. Treatment is by wide local excision of the disease and the associated scar, to reduce the risk of recurrence (reported rate is over 10%).

Inguinal endometriosis presents as a painful mass. Overlying skin changes and cyclic symptoms vary. Endometriosis has been found in hernia sacs, in old inguinal scars and in the inguinal lymphatics. Treatment is by inguinal exploration and excision.

Nervous system

The most common sites are the nerves in the pelvis. When sciatic pain occurs in relation to the menstrual cycle, it should suggest the presence of endometriosis. Involvement of the obturator nerve may produce pain and weakness in the proximal muscles of the thigh. The treatment is exploration and excision of endometriosis and fibrosis surrounding the nerve.

In men

Endometriosis has been reported in men undergoing treatment for prostate cancer by excision, and orchidectomy and high-dose oestrogen therapy. The reduction in testosterone after removal of the testicles augmented by oestrogen therapy could account for these cases.

CHAPTER 9

Recurrent endometriosis

Even with good medical and surgical management, endometriosis is a progressive disease that tends to recur after treatment. The reasons for this are still unclear, but it may be due to:

- evolution of lesions
- persistence due to lack of recognition of visible, but subtle, lesions
- lack of identification of subperitoneal lesions
- incomplete excision at laparoscopy or laparotomy.

The diagnosis of recurrence is based on the symptoms and signs, and physical examination, together with transvaginal ultrasonography, MRI or CA-125 immunoassay, if appropriate.

After laparotomy

In 1953, Meigs noted the recurrence of symptoms in 7% (15/215) of patients, but did not re-operate on any patient. Punnonen, in the largest study published, observed a recurrence rate of 15% in a 6–10 year follow-up of 903 patients surgically treated for the disease. Wheeler and Malinak, in a classic study of 423 patients, documented a 10% recurrence rate; the annual recurrence rate varied from 1% (first year) to 14% in the eighth year, with a cumulative rate of 14% at 3 years and 40% at 5 years.

After laparoscopic surgery

Fayez and colleagues reported on 162 women with infertility and stage I or stage II endometriosis: 82 had laparoscopic excision and 80 received danazol, 600 mg/day, for 6 months. Follow-up laparoscopy 1 year later revealed that the disease had recurred in 4% (3/82) and 9% (7/80) of the two groups, respectively. These findings confirm that postoperative danazol does not reduce the risk of recurrence.

Redwine and colleagues demonstrated a 5-year cumulative recurrence rate of 10% among 359 women with endometriosis (stages I–IV), who were treated by laparoscopic excision and followed up for 2 years. Canis and colleagues found 10% of patients had persistent lesions after excision of deep ovarian endometriomas.

After medical treatment

Evers and colleagues found the recurrence rate after medical therapy to be 29–51%. The difference between various recurrence rates is due to the length of time before follow-up, and diagnosis of recurrence (either by the patient's symptoms, laparoscopy, with or without histological confirmation). Evers advised against second-look laparoscopy during medical therapy.

After hysterectomy and bilateral salpingo-oophorectomy

Recurrence after radical surgery is thought to be rare. In 1970, Ranney reported no recurrences when oestrogen replacement was not given, and 3% when it was. In 1973, Gray reported no recurrences when hormones were not given and 20% if they were. Importantly, most recurrences included bowel involvement.

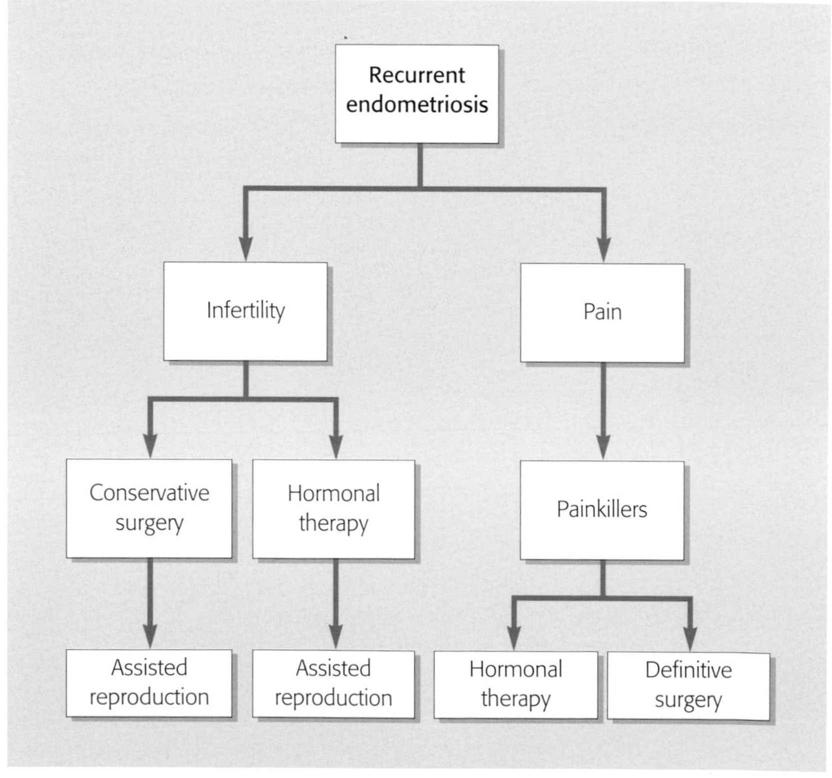

Figure 9.1 Treatment options for recurrent endometriosis.

Causes of recurrence

Ovarian remnant syndrome occurs if the ovary is not completely removed at the time of the surgery, possibly because of dense pelvic adhesions to the pelvic side-wall, or to the bladder and ureters. The most common presentation of this syndrome is pain unrelieved by analgesics. Measurement of FSH is useful in making the diagnosis, but this also relies on histological confirmation of ovarian tissue obtained at the time of the operation.

Steroid receptors and endometriosis. A study by Metzer and colleagues showed a difference between receptors in normal endometrium and those in endometrial implants. Therefore, hormonal medications that work on normal endometrium (e.g. oral contraceptives) might not work in endometriosis. This may explain a poor response following hormone treatment.

Extrapelvic endometriosis has been reported in several postmenopausal women, who may or may not have had endometriosis at an earlier age. In these cases, the most common sites for the disease are the urinary tract and bowel.

Management

The methods of treating recurrent endometriosis are outlined in Figure 9.1.

CHAPTER 10

Adenomyosis

Adenomyosis is the invasion of the endometrial glands and/or stroma within the myometrium. It is more common in women who have had children rather than those who have not, and generally appears between the ages of 40 and 70 years.

Though often called endometriosis interna, endometriosis and adenomyosis are present simultaneously in fewer than one in four patients. The glands appear histologically similar to the basalis part of the endometrium, so they do not usually undergo the proliferative and secretory changes associated with cyclic ovarian hormone production. The diagnosis rests on finding these glands beneath the endometrial surface, within the uterine muscle layer.

Prevalence

Published material gives a widely variable prevalence. Adenomyosis is usually diagnosed incidently by the pathologist examining surgical specimens, so prevalence relates directly to such research. More than 60% of women in the 40–70-year age range may be affected.

Pathogenesis

As with endometriosis, the pathogenesis of adenomyosis remains unknown. The accepted hypothesis is that high oestrogen levels stimulate hyperplasia of the basalis layer of the endometrium, thus causing the barrier between the endometrium and myometrium to break down. The stroma and subsequently the glands begin to invade the myometrium along the path of least resistance; in most cases, this growth is adjacent to lymphatic and vascular channels. The cause of this down-growth could be a mechanical factor, such as childbirth or curettage. Chronic inflammation could also damage the endometrial and myometrial borders and facilitate endometrial down-growth.

Oestrogen receptors are always found in adenomyomatous tissue, though in reduced quantity compared with normal myometrium. If progesterone receptors are present, they are found in fewer numbers than in normal endometrium.

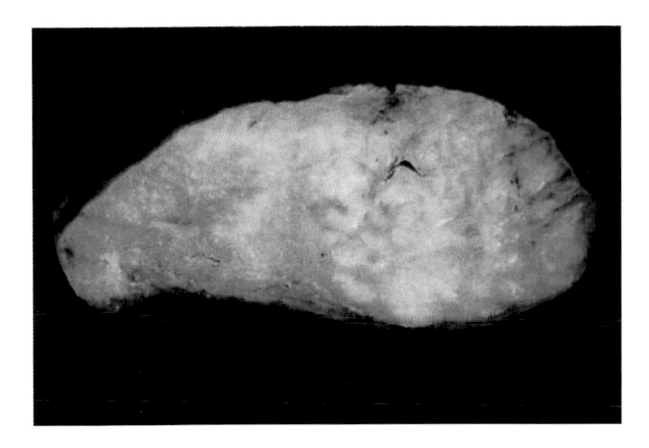

Figure 10.1 Cut surface of a uterus showing diffuse and distinct adenomyosis. Reproduced with permission from Nezhat CR *et al.*, eds. *Endometriosis: Advanced Management and Surgical Techniques.* New York: Springer-Verlag, 1995.

Pathology

The two forms of adenomyosis are:

- distinct
- diffuse (most common).

Both the anterior and posterior walls of the uterus can be involved, though the disease is more likely to occur in the posterior wall. In the diffused form, there are no encapsulated areas of adenomyosis. The uterus is enlarged asymmetrically up to three times its normal size (less than the size it would be at 14 weeks' gestation). The cut surface has a spongy appearance and protrudes convexly (Figure 10.1).

The standard criterion for diagnosis is the finding of endometrial glands and stroma 3 mm or more from the basalis layer of the endometrium. Histologically, the glands exhibit an inactive or proliferative pattern.

Endometrial hyperplasia is common. In the rare cases where adenocarcinoma develops, the diagnosis can be extremely difficult. Symptoms are lacking and there is no diagnostic tool other than hysterectomy; Woodruff *et al.* have, however, found malignant cells in cervical smears from such patients. There have also been various reports of a high prevalence of adenomyosis in patients with endometrial cancer, but there are no data to suggest that adenomyosis predisposes women to malignant degeneration.

Clinical diagnosis

Most women with adenomyosis are asymptomatic. Some women in their 40s and 50s show the classic symptoms of secondary dysmenorrhoea and menorrhagia, which become more severe as the disease progresses. Occasionally, the patient complains of dyspareunia felt deep in the pelvis and midline in location.

On pelvic examination, the uterus is globular. In premenopausal women, it may be tender to the touch immediately before and after menstruation.

Investigations

Myometrial biopsy remains the gold standard for a diagnosis without a hysterectomy specimen (Figure 10.2). These biopsies can be obtained via laparotomy, laparoscopy or hysteroscopy, and techniques are continually improving. Unfortunately, many cases can be overlooked unless the disease is extensive. McCausland used a 27 F operative hysteroscope and took biopsies of the posterior wall with a 5 mm loop electrode in 90 patients. This study confirmed the efficacy of the procedure, with no complications of either bleeding or perforation. However, this technique is contraindicated in postmenopausal women, because of the high risk of perforating the thin uterine wall.

Ultrasound. Both transabdominal and transvaginal ultrasound have been used to diagnose adenomyosis, with a positive predictive value of 70%.

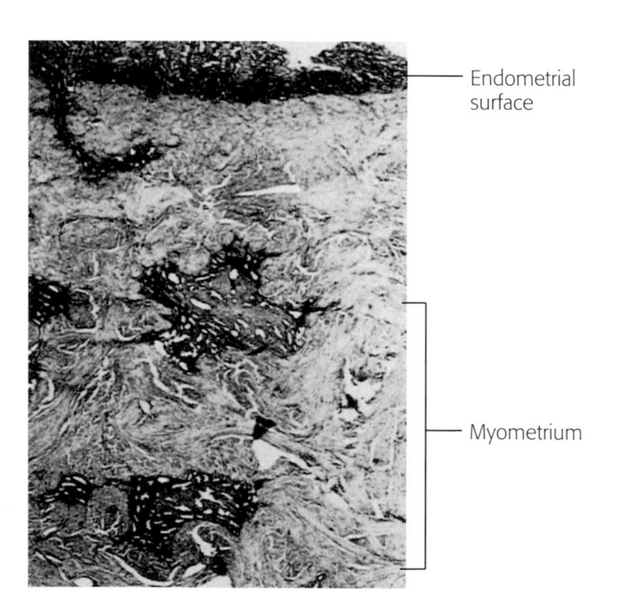

Figure 10.2 Myometrial biopsy showing islands of endometrial tissue deep within the myometrium. Reproduced with permission from Janovski NA *et al. Atlas of Gynecological and Obstetric Diagnostic Histopathology*. New York: McGraw-Hill, 1967.

MRI is the ideal procedure. In expert hands, it is most sensitive and can differentiate adenomyosis from the presence of fibroids.

Hysteroscopy. On rare occasions, visualization of a small endometrial diverticulum during hysteroscopy can raise suspicion of adenomyosis.

Hysterosalpingography is poor for confirming or excluding a diagnosis of adenomyosis.

CA-125. Data from a study comparing CA-125 levels in patients with adenomyosis with those of patients with fibroids are contradictory. Theoretically, if ectopic endometrium produces CA-125, the serum levels in patients with adenomyosis should be increased, and therapy should lower the CA-125 concentration.

Treatment of adenomyosis

Hysterectomy is the definitive treatment if the patient's age and parity permit. Pre-operative endometrial sampling should be carried out to exclude malignancy. The route of hysterectomy (abdominal or vaginal) and whether bilateral oophorectomy is required is determined by age and other surgical conditions.

Endometrial resection. Through advances in diagnostic imaging, conservative interventions such as endometrial ablation or endometrial resection have been proposed. Simple endometrial ablation is not able to resolve adenomyosis because, by definition, it is too deep. Ablation must go much deeper or endomyometrial resection or myometrial excision has to be performed.

Levonorgestrel-releasing IUD. Menorrhagia associated with adenomyosis has recently been successfully treated with an IUD that releases levonorgestrel.

Medical treatment of adenomyosis consists of GnRH agonists, danazol, cyclic hormones and prostaglandin synthetase inhibitors for pain and abnormal uterine bleeding. Two patients receiving GnRH therapy carried a pregnancy to full term.

CHAPTER 11

The doctor/patient partnership

There have been many references, in the many thousands of papers published about the disease, to the puzzle that is endometriosis. For those with the disease, the fact that it is 'a riddle wrapped in a mystery inside an enigma' (as one specialist wrote) will not bring comfort. Their hope is that a solution will be found that will eradicate the pain and suffering they endure while the disease is present.

Because of its nature, a diagnosis of endometriosis will be the start of a long-term, on-going relationship with a family physician and gynaecologist. It is important that the professionals establish this at the earliest stage, showing interest and concern in the woman and her general well-being. You have to obtain the essential facts, and explain both the illness and the treatment options in a way that your patient understands, so that she appreciates the choices open to her. Encourage questions and suggest ways that your patient can find out more about her condition (e.g. recommend books or self-help groups).

Your patient will probably want to know about:

- pain and discomfort that she might experience (over and above that of the disease itself)
- the risks of the proposed treatments, including anything that might affect her ability to have a child
- side-effects
- how much time is involved in treatment
- whether she will need to take time off work
- whether she will be incapacitated and need help with her family.

If the woman wants a second opinion, encourage her with the name of another specialist in endometriosis. She needs to be reassured that treatment suggested is appropriate. This is especially important if she has been told she must have a hysterectomy, or if nothing further can be done to treat the disease.

Having tried conventional treatment it may, in some cases, be useful to suggest coping strategies to deal with the primary symptom of pain: gentle heat applied to the abdomen of lower back, non-jarring exercise such as swimming and walking, acupuncture, physiotherapy, reflexology, using relaxation and visualization tapes. Encourage the woman to help herself, to enter into a partnership of treatment.

Useful addresses

The National Endometriosis Society
Suite 50
Westminster Palace Gardens
1–7 Artillery Row
London SW1P 1RL
UK
Telephone: +44 (0)171 222 2781 (administration)
+44 (0)171 222 2776 (national helpline 14.00–17.00 Mondays and Tuesdays, plus 19.00–22.00 daily)
Fax: +44 (0)171 222 2786

Endometriosis Association International Headquarters
8585 N 76th Place
Milwaukee WI 53223
USA
Telephone: +1 (414) 355 2200
Telephone: (toll-free N America) +1 800 992 3636
Fax: +1 (414) 355 6065
E-mail: endo@endometriosisassn.org
Website: www.Endometriosisassn.org

Key references

GENERAL

Adashi EY, Rock JA, Rosenwaks Z, eds. *Reproductive Endocrinology, Surgery and Technology.* Vol 2. Philadelphia: Lippincott-Raven, 1996.

Haney AF. Endometriosis. In: Lobo RA, Mishell DR, Paulson RJ *et al.*, eds. *Mishell's Textbook of Infertility, Contraception and Reproductive Endocrinology.* 4th ed. Oxford: Blackwell Scientific Fourth Edition, 1997:653–5.

Nezhat CR, Berger GS, Nezhat FR *et al.*, eds. *Endometriosis, Advanced Management and Surgical Techniques.* New York: Springer-Verlag, 1995.

Olive DL, *Endometriosis. Obstet Gynecol Clin N Am.* Vol 24, No 2. Philadelphia: WB Saunders Co, 1997.

Shaw RW, ed. *Advances in Reproductive Endocrinology: Endometriosis.* Vol 1. Carnforth: Parthenon Publishing, 1990.

NATURAL HISTORY

American Fertility Society. Classification of endometriosis. *Fertil Steril* 1979,32:633.

American Fertility Society: Revised classification of endometriosis. *Fertil Steril* 1985,43:351.

Mahmood TA, Templeton A. *Prevalence and Genesis of Endometriosis. Hum Reprod* 1991;6(4):544–9.

Hadfield R, Mardon H, Barlow D, Kennedy S. Delay in the diagnosis of endometriosis: a survey of women from the USA and the UK. *Hum Reprod* 1996;11(4):878–80.

American Society for Reproductive Medicine. Revised American Society for Reproductive Medicine classification of endometriosis. *Fertil Steril* 1997;67(5):817.

Halme J, Sahakian V. Endometriosis: pathophysiology and presentation. In: Keye WR, Chang RJ, Rebar RW *et al.*, eds. *Infertility – Evaluation and Treatment.* Philadelphia: WB Saunders Co, 1995:496–508.

Van der Linden PJQ. Theories on the pathogenesis of endometriosis. *Hum Reprod* 1996;11(Suppl 3):53–65.

Vessey MP, Villard-Mackintosh L, Painter R. Epidemiology of endometriosis in women attending family planning clinics. *BMJ* 1993;306:182–4.

TREATMENT

Brosens I. Pathophysiology and medical treatment of endometriosis associated infertility. In: Seibel MM, ed. *Infertility: A Comprehensive Text.* Stamford: Appleton & Lange, 1997:189–202.

Corson SL. *Endometriosis: The Enigmatic Disease.* Durant, Canada: Essential Medical Information Systems, 1992.

Dlugi AM, Miller JD, Knittle J. Lupron depot (leuprolide acetate for depot suspension) in the treatment of endometriosis: a randomized, placebo-controlled, double-blind study. Lupron Study Group. *Fertil Steril* 1990;54(3):419–27.

Hesla J, Rock J. Endometriosis. In: Rock JA, Thompson JD, eds. *Te Linde's Operative Gynaecology.* 8th ed. New York: Lippincott-Raven, 1997:585.

Kim AH, Adamson GD. Results of surgical therapy for endometriosis. In: Olive DL, ed. *Operative Techniques in Gynecologic Surgery: Surgery for Endometriosis.* Vol 2 (2). Philadelphia: WB Saunders Co, 1997:122–9.

INFERTILITY

Nasseri A, Copperman AB. Endometriosis and its effects on assisted reproduction technologies: a review. *Assisted Reprod Rev* 1997;7:71–6.

Oosterlynck DJ, Cornille FJ, Waer M *et al.* Women with endometriosis show a defect in natural killer activity resulting in a decreased cytotoxicity to autologous endometrium. *Fertil Steril* 1991;56:45–51.

Rizk B, Aboulghar M, Smitz J *et al.* The role of vascular endothelial growth factor and interleukins in the pathogenesis of severe ovarian hyperstimulation syndrome. *Hum Reprod Update* 1997;3:255–66.

Rizk B, Aksel S, Helvacioglu A. Gamete intrafallopian transfer in patients with pelvic endometriosis. *Gynecol Obstet Reprod Med* 1995;1:124–6.

Schenken RS. Treatment of human infertility: the special case of endometriosis. In: Adashi EY, Rock JA, Rosenwaks Z, eds. *Reproductive Endocrinology, Surgery and Technology.* Vol 2. Philadelphia: Lippincott-Raven, 1996.

Society of Assisted Reproductive Technology and Centers for Disease Control. Assisted reproductive technology success rates – national summary and fertility clinic reports, Vol 2 Central US, 1995. Atlanta: RESOLVE, 1997.

ADENOMYOSIS

Azziz R. Adenomyosis: current perspectives. *Obstet Gynecol Clin N Am* 1989;16:221–35.

Droegemueller W. Endometriosis and adenomyosis. In: Mishell DR, Stenchever MA, Droegemueller W *et al.*, eds. *Comprehensive Gynecology.* St Louis: Mosby, 1997:18.

Jen SW, Lim-Tan SK, Wee D *et al.* The clinical significance of adenomyosis and its relation to fertility. *Advances in Fertility and Sterility series.* Vol 5. London: Parthenon Publishing, 1987:207–12.

Index

adenomyosis 15, 64–7
adhesiolysis 4, 32, 41, 44
adhesions 5, 15, 18, 22, 24, 25, 30, 32, 43, 45, 50, 63
adnexal masses 4, 28, 42
age as risk factor 10
alcohol as risk factor 10, 13
amenorrhoea 4, 36
anovulation 4, 23, 24, 48
assisted reproduction technology 52–5, 62

blebs 4, 32
body fat distribution 10, 14

cancer 8, 14, 16, 60, 65, 67
classification 17–18
contraceptives as risk factor 10, 12, 13

diagnosis 7, 27–34, 41, 65–6
  differential 30
dioxins 10–11, 14
dizygotic 4, 10
dyschezia 4, 27, 28, 29
dysmenorrhoea 4, 27, 28, 29, 38, 45, 65
dyspareunia 4, 27, 28, 29, 38, 45, 66
dysuria 4, 29, 58

endometrial atrophy 4, 36
endometrioma 4, 18, 29, 32–3, 41, 42, 43, 50, 62
endometriosis scores 4, 18
environmental risk factors 10–11
epidemiology 7–14
expectant management 48, 49
extrapelvic endometriosis 56–60, 63

fecundity rate 4, 22, 47, 52–5
fibroids 8, 67

gastrointestinal tract endometriosis 41, 56–7, 63
GnRH 4, 35, 36, 37, 38–9, 48, 59, 67

gynaecological surgery 7, 8–9

haematuria 4, 29
heredity as risk factor 9, 10, 27, 28
hirsutism 4, 36
history taking 27, 28
hormonal therapy 35–40, 58, 62
  side-effects 36, 37, 38
hormone replacement therapy (HRT) 10, 27, 44
hormones as risk factor 10
hypermenorrhoea 4, 29
hyperplasia 4, 8, 64, 65
hyperprolactinaemia 4, 23, 24
hysterectomy 7, 8–9, 41, 43–4, 62, 63, 67, 68

immunoassays 28, 34, 61, 67
immunological abnormalities 23, 25–6
implantation 4, 17, 18, 26
implantation theory 15–16
induction theory 16, 17
infertility 5, 7, 22–6, 27, 28, 29, 35, 42, 45, 61
  pelvic factors 22, 25
  treatment 47–51
  see also assisted reproduction technology
in situ development 16–17
IUDs as risk factor 10, 12

laparoscopy 5, 7, 27, 28, 31–2, 35, 41–3, 46, 47, 48, 50–1, 61–2, 66
laparotomy 5, 50–1, 61, 66

macrophages 4, 23, 24
medical treatment 35–40, 47–8, 48–51, 62, 67
menstrual history 10, 11–13, 28, 29
mesothelium 4, 19
metaplasia 4, 16, 17
monozygotic 4, 10
MRI 28, 32–4, 61, 67

neurectomy 41, 45–6

oestradiol 4, 36
oligomenorrhoea 4, 29
oophorectomy 4, 41, 59, 62, 67
osteoporosis 14, 38, 39, 44
ovarian cysts 17–18, 30
ovulation disorders 23, 24–5

partnership in treatment 68–9
pathogenesis 15–17
pelvic pain 7, 8, 23, 25, 27, 28, 29, 30, 38, 40, 42, 45–6
peritoneal fluid 4
  abnormalities 22–4
prevalence 5, 7–9
progestogens 35, 36, 37, 39, 44
prostaglandins 4, 20, 23
psychological impact 4, 68

race as risk factor 9, 10
rectal bleeding 29, 57
recurrent endometriosis 61–3
remnant theory 16, 17, 61, 63
reproductive history 10, 11–13
retrograde menstruation 4
risk factors 9–14, 27

sites 15, 56–60
smoking as risk factor 10, 14
spontaneous abortion 23, 26
stages 19–21
superovulation 4, 53
surgical treatment 41–6
  for infertility 47, 48–51
  radical 43–4, 62
symptoms and signs 27–9

tubal distortion 7, 13, 18, 22, 23, 25

ultrasonography 28, 32, 34, 61, 66
urinary tract endometriosis 41, 57–8, 63
uterine fibroids 4, 14